The Assessment
of Psychoses

The Assessment of Psychoses

A PRACTICAL HANDBOOK

Edited by

Thomas R.E. Barnes

Professor of Clinical Psychiatry,
Horton Hospital, Epsom, UK

and

Hazel E. Nelson

Consultant Psychologist,
Horton Hospital, Epsom, UK

CHAPMAN & HALL MEDICAL

London · Glasgow · Weinheim · New York · Tokyo · Melbourne · Madras

Published by Chapman & Hall, 2–6 Boundary Row, London SE1 8HN

Chapman & Hall, 2–6 Boundary Row, London SE1 8HN, UK

Blackie Academic & Professional, Wester Cleddens Road, Bishopbriggs, Glasgow G64 2NZ, UK

Chapman & Hall GmbH, Pappelallee 3, 69469 Weinheim, Germany

Chapman & Hall USA, One Penn Plaza, 41st Floor, New York NY 10119, USA

Chapman & Hall Japan, ITP Japan, Kyowa Building, 3F, 2-2-1, Hirakawacho, Chiyoda-ku, Tokyo 102, Japan

Chapman & Hall Australia, Thomas Nelson Australia, 102 Dodds Street, South Melbourne, Victoria 3205, Australia

Chapman & Hall India, R. Seshadri, 32 Second Main Road, CIT East, Madras 600 035, India

First edition 1994

© 1994 Thomas R.E. Barnes and Hazel Nelson

Printed at Alden Press Limited, Oxford and Northampton, Great Britain

ISBN 0 412 53590 4

A catalogue record for this book is available from the British Library

Library of Congress Catalog Number is available

∞ Printed on permanent acid-free text paper, manufactured in accordance with ANSI/NISO Z39.48-1992 and ANSI/NISO Z39.48-1984 (Permanence of Paper)

Contents

CONTENTS

Contributors

Thomas R.E. Barnes, Horton Hospital, Long Grove Road, Epsom, Surrey KT19 8PZ, UK

David A. Curson, Medical Director, Medical Wing, The Royal Masonic Hospital, Ravenscourt Park, London W6 0TN, UK

John Cutting, Consultant Psychiatrist, The Bethlem Royal Hospital, Monks Orchard Road, Beckenham, Kent BR3 3BX, UK

David Baldwin, The Academic Department of Psychiatry, Saint Mary's Hospital, Praed Street, London W2 1NY, UK

Janis Flint, Department of Psychiatry, Charing Cross Hospital, Fulham Palace Road, London W6 8RF, UK

Philippa Garety, Lecturer in Psychology, Institute of Psychiatry, De Crespigny Park, Denmark Hill, London SE5 8AF, UK

Keith Hawton, Consultant Psychiatrist and Senior Lecturer, Department of Psychiatry, Warneford Hospital, Oxford OX3 7JX, UK

Professor John M. Kane, Chairman, Department of Psychiatry, Hillside Hospital, P.O. Box 38, Glen Oaks, New York 10461, USA

Shôn Lewis, Senior Lecturer, Department of Psychiatry, Charing Cross Hospital, Fulham Palace Road, London W6 8RF, UK

Peter Liddle, Senior Lecturer, Hammersmith Hospital, Du Cane Road, London W12 0HS, UK

Brigid MacCarthy, Psychologist, Ealing Hospital, Saint Bernard's Wing, Uxbridge Road, Southall, Middlesex UB1 3EU, UK

Robin G. McCreadie, Director of Clinical Research, Crichton Royal Hospital, Dumfries DG1 4TG, UK

Deirdre Montgomery, The Academic Department of Psychiatry, Saint Mary's Hospital, Praed Street, London W2 1NY, UK

Stuart A. Montgomery, The Academic Department of Psychiatry, Saint Mary's Hospital, Praed Street, London W2 1NY, UK

Hazel E. Nelson, Horton Hospital, Long Grove Road, Epsom, Surrey KT19 8PZ, UK

Christos Pantelis, Cognitive Neuropsychiatry Research Unit, Mental Health Research Institute, Private Bag, 3, Parkville, Victoria 3052, Australia

George Patton, Saint James House, 108, Hampstead Road, Bloomsbury, London NW1 2LT, UK

Robert Pugh, Shenley Hospital, Shenley, Radlett, Hertfordshire WD5 9HB, UK

Robert Sharrock, Lecturer in Clinical Psychology, IARC Ash Ridge, 17m, Portland Place, London W1N 3AF, UK

Sheila Stayte, Shenley Hospital, Shenley, Radlett, Hertfordshire WD5 9HB, UK

CONTRIBUTORS

Kate H. Tress, Saint James House, 108, Hampstead Road, Bloomsbury, London NW1 2LT, UK

Simon Wessely, Institute of Psychiatry, De Crespigny Park, Denmark Hill, London SE5 8AF, UK

Richard Whittington, IARC Ash Ridge, 17m, Portland Place, London W1N 3AF, UK

Til Wykes, IARC Ash Ridge, 17m, Portland Place, London W1N 3AF, UK

Preface

The prime aim of this book is to present the reader with systematic information on the major rating scales available for the assessment of the main areas of psychopathology, behaviour and functioning in patients with psychotic illness. For each area, the major rating scales available are reviewed by psychiatrists and psychologists who are recognized specialists in their fields and who have extensive practical experience in the scales' uses. Practical details are given, together with the more theoretical details of reliability, validity and utility, so that both clinicians and researchers can select the most appropriate scales for their particular purposes.

We are grateful to all the contributors for their hard work, for agreeing to comply with the standard format for each of the chapters and for their insights into the assessment of the various aspects of psychotic illness. We would like to thank Sue Benthall and Janet Grimshaw for their patience in typing and re-typing chapters, and Farrand Press for its support and good humour throughout all stages of the preparation of this book. We hope it will prove a useful resource for psychologists, psychiatrists, nurses and others involved in the care, treatment and investigation of those with psychotic illness.

Thomas Barnes
Hazel Nelson
September 1993

ERRATUM

We very much regret that, in the first printing, this table was omitted from chapter one, where it is referred to on page one.

TABLE 1. *Diagnostic criteria used in original papers published in three journals in 1988.*

| Criteria | British Journal of Psychiatry* | | | | Acta Psychiatrica Scandinavica | | | | Archives of General Psychiatry | | | |
| | Schizophrenia | | Affective Illness | | Schizophrenia | | Affective Illness | | Schizophrenia | | Affective Illness | |
	N	%	N	%	N	%	N	%	N	%	N	%
DSM III	3	15	5	33	10	47	20	57	13	52	8	44
RDC	6	30	2	13	5	24	9	26	11	44	9	50
Feighner	7	35	2	13	1	5	1	3	-	-	-	-
ICD	2	10	5	33	4	19	4	11	1	4	-	-
PSE	2	10	-	-	1	5	-	-	-	-	-	-
Newcastle	-	-	1	8	-	-	1	3	-	-	1	6
Total	20	100	15	100	21	100	35	100	25	100	18	100

*Significant minority with no criteria given for diagnosis.

1. The Assessment of Psychopathology for Diagnosis

Robin G. McCreadie

If patients in different countries or in different centres in the same country were given the same diagnostic label defined in different ways, then it would be impossible to evaluate published research on aetiology, treatment and prognosis. We need, therefore, clear concise diagnostic criteria, understandable to psychiatrists and applicable to patients wherever they are.

Table I shows the range of diagnostic criteria for schizophrenia and affective illness used in original papers published in 1988 in three eminent psychiatric journals, *The British Journal of Psychiatry, Acta Psychiatrica Scandinavica* and *Archives of General Psychiatry*. It can be seen that in the United States only two sets of criteria are used, DSM III and Research Diagnostic Criteria, whilst the range of criteria in the United Kingdom is wider. Scandinavian practice is different again, but veers more towards the United States. This chapter considers the advantages and disadvantages of these different criteria.

The Process of Assessment

A diagnosis cannot be made without detailed knowledge of the patient. This is best obtained through direct contact with the patient, either through an open or structured interview. Some diagnostic scales can be applied to case notes, but very considerable detail would be necessary for this to be successful.

Once the research worker has such detailed knowledge the time taken to complete the diagnostic scales described below is usually measured in minutes.

The Assessment Procedures

Research Diagnostic Criteria (RDC)
(Spitzer et al., 1978; Endicott and Spitzer, 1978)

The Research Diagnostic Criteria were developed to enable research investigators to apply a consistent set of criteria for subjects with functional psychiatric illness. The purpose is to obtain relatively homogeneous groups. Subjects who do not meet any of the criteria, but have some evidence of psychiatric disturbance are classified as "other psychiatric disorder". The authors believe it is better to avoid false positives than false negatives.

The main source of data for making diagnostic judgements is direct examination of the patient, either by a focused clinical interview or by the structured interview guide and rating scale called the Schedule for Affective Disorders and Schizophrenia (SADS). A lifetime version of SADS can be used when it is unlikely the subject is in a current episode of illness. RDC can also be used with detailed case record material. All diagnoses are judged no/probable/definite. Since "probable" implies more than 50 per cent certainty, it should not be used for two mutually exclusive diagnoses for the same episode of illness.

All conditions in RDC can be diagnosed only where there is no likely known organic aetiology for the symptoms.

The RDC includes the following definitions of clinical terms.

Schizophrenia

There are three main sets of criteria, all of which must be fulfilled. The first is a "menu" of symptoms present during the active phase of the illness; two must be present for "definite" and one for "probable" schizophrenia. The majority are either Schneiderian "first rank" or Crow's "positive" symptoms. The second main criterion specifies the illness must have lasted at least two weeks. There is no other time limit, and thus RDC avoids limiting the diagnosis to cases with a chronic or deteriorating course. The third criterion stipulates that during the active phase the patient did not meet the criteria for manic or depressive syndrome.

Affective Disorder

Manic Disorder   There are five main sets of criteria, all of which must be fulfilled. The first describes a change in mood, the second a "menu" of symptoms, the third a change in social functioning, the fourth a duration of manic features of at least one week, and the fifth a list of exclusion symptoms which suggest schizophrenia.

Major Depressive Disorder   Here there are six sets of criteria: a change in mood, a menu of symptoms, a duration of at least one week, a change in social functioning, exclusion symptoms of schizophrenia, and exclusion of schizophrenia (residual type).

Major Depressive Disorder has a number of sub-types of which Psychotic Major Depressive Disorder (presence of delusions or hallucinations) and Endogenous Major Depressive Disorder (which describes two menus of largely biological symptoms) are especially useful in the diagnosis of functional psychoses.

Schizo-affective Disorder (manic or depressed type)

This category is for patients who have had an episode of illness that fulfils criteria from the menu of symptoms of either mania or depression, but who also have at least one from a menu of symptoms suggesting schizophrenia *concurrent* with the manic or depressive syndrome. The authors believe this category helps "purify" the samples of schizophrenia and affective disorder.

Reliability and validity

Inter-rater and test-retest reliability of the RDC categories was tested with psychiatric inpatients in three studies (Spitzer *et al.*, 1978). The first two studies involved joint interviews where one rater conducted the interview and the other observed. Both made independent ratings. In the first study (68 patients rated) the kappa coefficient of agreement for schizophrenia was 0.80, for manic disorder 0.82, for major depressive disorder 0.88 and for schizoaffective disorder, depressed type 0.86. The coefficients in the second study (150 patients with affective illness rated) were 0.98 for manic disorder, 0.90 for major depressive disorder, and 0.85 for schizoaffective disorder, depressed type. In the test-retest reliability study 60 patients were rated twice within a day or two. The kappa coefficient for schizophrenia was 0.65, manic disorder 0.82, major depressive disorder 0.90, schizoaffective disorder manic type 0.79, and schizoaffective disorder depressed type 0.73. The results of these three studies indicate that the reliability of the RDC categories is high, even under test-retest conditions where a much lower reliability is expected.

Utility
This classification is best used if the research investigator wishes to include schizophrenics and patients with affective illness with *short lived* episodes. It also clearly separates these two conditions from schizo-affective psychoses.

Diagnostic and Statistical Manual of Mental Disorders (Third Edition) (DSM III)
Diagnostic and Statistical Manual of Mental Disorders (Third Edition) - Revised (DSM III-R)
(Published by the American Psychiatric Association, 1980 and 1987 respectively)

This set of diagnostic criteria was produced for the American Psychiatric Association by a task force, selected because of members' special interest in various aspects of diagnosis, and chaired by Dr Spitzer. DSM III was compiled with the principal goals of usefulness, reliability and acceptability to clinicians and researchers. It is "atheoretical" with regard to aetiology except for those disorders for which a pathophysiological process is well established.

DSM III and RDC have many similarities. DSM III includes the following technical terms:

Schizophrenia

In DSM III six main criteria must be fulfilled. As with RDC, the first is a menu of first rank and/or positive symptoms of which one must be present; the second stipulates a deterioration in level of functioning, and the third a duration of continuous signs of illness for *at least 6 months* at some time during the person's life; the fourth excludes depressive or manic syndrome; the fifth stipulates the illness must start before the age of *45 years* and the sixth that there is no organic mental disorder or mental retardation.

In DSM III-R the main changes are, firstly, that schizo-affective disorder is ruled out (see below); secondly, if there is a history of autistic disorder, the additional diagnosis of schizophrenia is made only if delusions or hallucinations are also prominent; and thirdly, the age limit of 45 years is dropped – but "late onset" must be specified if the illness begins after that age.

Paranoid Disorders

DSM III unlike RDC has a category for patients with persecutory delusions, but no other features from the menu of first rank/positive symptoms.

Schizophreniform Disorder

Criteria are identical to schizophrenia with the exception that the duration of disturbance is less than 6 months, but more than 2 weeks. In DSM III-R the characteristic psychotic symptoms in the active phase must have lasted at least 1 week.

Major Affective Disorders

Manic episode   In DSM III, there are five main criteria: a change in mood; a duration of at least 1 week of at least three symptoms taken from a menu of seven; no preceding or subsequent mood incongruent delusions or hallucinations or bizarre behaviour; schizophrenia, schizophreniform disorder and paranoid disorder have been ruled out; organic brain disorder has been ruled out. DSM III-R has an additional criterion of social deterioration.

Major depressive episode   Here also in DSM III there are five very similar main criteria: a change in mood or loss of interest; a duration of at least 2 weeks of four symptoms from a menu of seven; no preceding or subsequent mood incongruent delusions, hallucinations or bizarre behaviour; no evidence of schizophrenia, schizophreniform disorder or paranoid disorder; no evidence of organic brain disorder.

There are two useful sub-categories, major depressive disorder with psychotic features (delusions, hallucinations or stupor (the latter is excluded in DSM III-R)) and major depressive disorder with melancholia (an emphasis on biological symptoms). DSM III-R highlights in this latter diagnosis previous good response to specific and adequate somatic antidepressant therapy (e.g. tricyclic antidepressants, ECT).

Schizo-affective Disorder

This category is retained in DSM III without diagnostic criteria. In DSM III-R there are four new criteria; the principal one is that at some time there is either a major depressive or a manic syndrome *concurrent* with symptoms from the "menu" criterion of schizophrenia.

Reliability and validity

Before official adoption of DSM-III a series of field trials was carried out (American Psychiatric Association, 1980). In all, 12 667 patients were assessed by 550 clinicians, 474 of whom were in 212 different facilities, using successive drafts of DSM-III. Criticisms resulted in numerous changes. The end result was that the great majority of participants, regardless of theoretical orientation, had a favourable response to DSM-III.

Inter-rater reliability was assessed by having pairs of clinicians make independent diagnostic judgements of several hundred patients. In two separate phases of DSM-III development kappa coefficients of agreement for schizophrenic disorders was 0.81 (60 patients rated) and 0.81 (77 patients rated); for major affective disorders 0.68 (98 patients rated) and 0.80 (89 patients rated); and for paranoid disorders 0.66 (four patients rated) and 0.75 (five patients rated).

Utility
DSM III and DSM III-R are very similar to RDC. DSM III criteria for schizophrenia are stricter than RDC and the disturbance has to have lasted longer (otherwise schizophreniform disorder is diagnosed). Also, for DSM III the patient must be aged under 45 at the time of first episode, though this latter criterion is dropped from DSM III-R. Like RDC, DSM III-R defines schizo-affective psychosis; this is not defined by DSM III.

The Feighner Criteria (also known as the St. Louis Criteria)
(Feighner et al., 1972)

These criteria are described by the authors as "a distillation of our clinical research experience, and of the experience of others". The diagnoses of schizophrenia and primary affective disorders are mutually exclusive. No effort has been made to sub-classify these illnesses, which are defined as below:

Schizophrenia
Four main criteria must be fulfilled: a chronic illness with at least 6 months of symptoms prior to index evaluation; no depressive or manic symptoms sufficient to qualify for affective disorder; delusions, hallucinations or verbal production that makes communication difficult; and three social or demographic features from a menu of five.

Primary Affective Disorders
Depression Three main criteria must be fulfilled: a change in mood; five symptoms for "definite" and four for "probable" from a menu of seven; and a duration of at least 1 month of symptoms with no pre-existing psychiatric conditions such as schizophrenia.

Mania Again there are three criteria: change in mood; three symptoms from a menu of six; and a duration of at least 2 weeks with no pre-existing psychiatric conditions. Patients with either depression or mania, but also with alteration of perceptions or thinking are classified as having an undiagnosed psychiatric disorder.

Reliability and validity
The classification is validated primarily by follow-up and family studies cited in the original publication. The authors also reported in the same paper a study of inter-rater reliability and validation of reliability with an 18 month follow-up study of 314 psychiatric emergency room patients as well as a 7 year follow-up of 87 psychiatric inpatients, each of whom was interviewed personally and systemati-

cally. Inter-rater agreement ranged from 86 to 95%. Validity as determined by correctly predicting diagnosis at follow-up was 93%.

Utility

In the diagnosis of schizophrenia there are two principal differences between the Feighner Criteria and DSM III and RDC. First, delusions and hallucinations are insufficiently described by the Feighner Criteria. Secondly, in the Feighner Criteria schizophrenia can be diagnosed without the presence of delusions or hallucinations. Thus the Feighner Criteria are less clear cut than either RDC or DSM III. Also, because Feighner can categorize as schizophrenic only those patients who have had symptoms for at least 6 months before the illness, it necessarily focuses on a more chronically disturbed group. Similarly, in the diagnosis of affective illness, the minimum time patients have to show symptoms is longer in Feighner than in RDC or DSM III.

International Classification of Diseases (Ninth Revision) – (ICD-9)
(Published by World Health Organization, 1978)

The psychiatric section of the International Classification of Diseases (ICD) uses criteria that are not uniform throughout. It follows predominantly descriptive lines, but aetiological and prognostic criteria are also used in some categories. There is a glossary of terms which is included to encourage uniformity of usage of descriptive and diagnostic terms.

    295 Schizophrenic psychoses
    296 Affective psychoses
    297 Paranoid states

These three categories give excellent but brief descriptions of the main disorder, and its subtypes.

Reliability and validity

Changes in the classification which resulted in ICD-8 and subsequently ICD-9 were carried out through a series of eight international seminars held between 1965 and 1972, each of which focused on a recognised problem area in psychiatric diagnosis. Psychiatrists from more than 40 countries participated. No formal attempt to assess reliability or validity was carried out before its introduction.

Utility

National statistics in the United Kingdom are compiled on the basis of ICD-9. As clinicians therefore use this classification as part of their everyday work, research studies using ICD-9 are likely to be acceptable and readily understandable to them. However, criticism expressed by the American Psychiatric Association in DSM III that many specific areas of classification are not sufficiently detailed for research use seems justified. ICD-10 will be accompanied by at least three sets of guidelines to cover diagnosis, research and the use of classification in general health care.

Present State Examination (PSE)
(Wing et al., 1974) (see also Chapter 6)

This is an interview technique which allows symptoms, defined in a glossary, to be elicited and reliably recorded. The interview can last from less than one to several hours. It assesses symptoms experienced or exhibited during the previous month only, so personality traits and social adjustment are excluded. Once rated, the symptoms can be grouped into syndromes on the basis of a computer programme (CATEGO). A clinical classification can be arrived at "with the final aim of making the eventual choice of a diagnostic term more reliable". The Catego classes are not intended to be recognized as a substitute for diagnosis.

The following classes can be derived in the examination of patients with functional psychoses:

Class S+ (central schizophrenic conditions)

Class M+ (manic and mixed affective psychoses)

Class D+ (depressive psychoses)

Class P+ (paranoid psychoses)

Class O+ (other psychoses – catatonic symptoms and/or behaviour indicative of hallucinations)

Reliability and validity
The interview schedule has a satisfactory degree of reliability and repeatability when raters have been adequately trained. For example, Wing and colleagues (1974) reported on 172 PSE interviews which were categorized by two psychiatrists on the basis of 77 simple descriptive categories. 116 interviews were inter-observer reliability comparisons and 56 repeatability comparisons. Complete agreement was obtained in 84% of cases. With regard to inter-observer reliability, there was 92% agreement for schizophrenia and 80% for psychotic depression.

Utility
The PSE should only be administered by trained raters (usually psychiatrists); training usually takes the form of a 1 week course run by experienced trainers. Another practical disadvantage of the PSE is that the interview may be lengthy and exhausting. The PSE is not primarily a diagnostic instrument. It arrives at categories which are similar to clinical diagnosis on the basis of an interview that excludes events previous to 1 month before the interview. Given these practical and theoretical limitations, it is not surprising that the PSE is little used as a diagnostic instrument.

Newcastle Diagnostic Index
(Carney et al., 1965)

This scale, which assesses depression, does not diagnose depression, but categorizes depressed patients into "endogenous" or "neurotic". Items which are used include adequate personality, weight loss, depressed psychomotor activity, anxiety and guilt. Each feature is weighted, and depending on the score a diagnosis of endogenous or reactive depression is made.

Reliability and validity
The differentiating features were arrived at through an investigation of 129 inpatient depressives treated with ECT. A factor analysis produced a bipolar factor corresponding to the distinction between endogenous and neurotic depression. Through multiple regression analysis the different factors received a weighting.

Utility
The scale does not diagnose depression, but may be used to select out endogenous depressives once the diagnosis is made.

Comparative Utility of the Diagnostic Instruments

If a research worker wishes a paper on functional psychosis to be published in a reputable American journal, it is clear patients must be diagnosed using either DSM III or RDC. There is now little to choose between the two since DSM III-R was introduced. In Britain ICD-9 and Feighner Criteria are also used, but they are less specific; in my opinion the American approach is correct. PSE and Newcastle Diagnostic Index, though used, are not designed as primarily diagnostic instruments.

References

American Psychiatric Association (1980). "Diagnostic and Statistical Manual of Mental Disorders". (3rd Edn). American Psychiatric Association, Washington DC.

American Psychiatric Association (1987). "Diagnostic and Statistical Manual of Mental Disorders". 3rd Edn, Revised. American Psychiatric Association, Washington DC.

Carney, M.W.P., Roth, M. and Garside, R.F. (1965). The diagnosis of depressive syndromes and the prediction of ECT response. *British Journal of Psychiatry,* **11**, 659-674.

Endicott, J. and Spitzer, R.L. (1978). A diagnostic interview. The schedule for affective disorders and schizophrenia. *Archives of General Psychiatry,* **35**, 837-844.

Feighner, J.P., Robins, E., Guze, S.B., Woodruff, R.A., Winokur, G. and Munoz, R. (1972). Diagnostic criteria for use in psychiatric research. *Archives of General Psychiatry,* **26**, 57-62.

Spitzer, R.L., Endicott, J. and Robins, E. (1978). Research diagnostic criteria: rationale and reliability. *Archives of General Psychiatry,* **35**, 773-782.

Wing, J.K., Cooper, J.E. and Sartorius, N. (1974). "The Measurement and Classification of

Psychiatric Symptoms". Cambridge University Press, Cambridge.

World Health Organisation (1978). Mental Disorders: Glossary and guide to their classification in accordance with the Ninth Revision of the International Classification of diseases. World Health Organisation, Geneva.

2. The Assessment of Change in Psychopathology

Kate H. Tress and George Patton

Scales for rating change in psychopathology have generally been developed to measure changes brought about by altering the treatment of a psychiatric disorder – particularly drug trials for new antipsychotic or antidepressant drugs. It would be possible to use very specific scales for a circumscribed set of symptoms and signs as described elsewhere in this book (e.g. thought disorder as reviewed in Chapter 4), but in a trial of a treatment it is important to see the effect of the treatment on the whole range of psychopathology. It is of limited use to find a drug that, for instance, eliminated auditory hallucinations but increased the strength of delusions and also induced severe depression.

The same considerations apply to monitoring treatment in the individual. Ideally the whole range of psychopathology should be rated, as any treatment administered may have subtle deleterious effects as well as obvious beneficial effects. It is then the task of the clinical team and the individual patient to weigh the positive against the negative effects of treatment. This is much more easily done if a complete record is kept and changes in psychopathology can be assessed in relation to changes in treatment. It also makes it easier to choose the appropriate treatment on any future occasion.

A third possible use of scales for rating psychopathology is in the monitoring of the natural history of the illness. If the course of an illness is monitored in this way over several months, new insights may be gained as to the nature of the illness and into the frequently encountered problem of a diagnosis not agreeing with one made on a second occasion. Fluctuations in the prominence of various diagnostically significant symptoms and signs, which might account for such discrepancies, could be readily identified by longtitudinal monitoring. Theoretical problems such as the origin and course of post-psychotic depression could also be addressed by such a method (e.g. Leff *et al.*, 1988).

The Process of Assessment

In the process of assessment the most usual sources of information available to the researcher wishing to study psychopathology are the patient's report of symptoms and the observation of their behaviour by trained mental health staff. The most commonly used scales draw, to a varying extent, on these two sources of information. Some, (e.g. PSE Change Rating Scale) utilize clinically based definitions while others (e.g. BPRS) contain items that are descriptive, not related to clinical concepts and not necessarily independent of other items. There are differences between scales in the extent to which psychotic symptoms (delusions and hallucinations) are viewed as occurring on a continuum of severity.

Although, for reasons described above, comprehensiveness is desirable in a scale rating change in psychopathology, in practice such a scale would be long and tedious to administer and score. This would have implications for the compliance of subjects (and raters!) who may be expected to undergo several repetitions of the procedure during a study. It may be necessary, in the interests of retaining the subject group (many of whom would have concentration and attention problems), to trade off comprehensiveness against brevity.

The Assessment Procedures

The Brief Psychiatric Rating Scale (BPRS)
(Overall and Gorham, 1962) (see also Chapters 3, 5 and 6)

The BPRS is intended as a quick and comprehensive rating scale for change in psychopathology developed from factor analysis of sets of items from two large scales (Lorr *et al.*, 1953, 1960). It takes 15-30 min to administer.

The scale consists of 16 "symptom constructs" each rated on a seven point scale of severity from "not present" to "extremely severe". The interviewer rates the subject on symptoms reported by the subject and behaviour noted during the interview. The authors suggest a standard interview with 3 min establishing rapport, 10 min non-directive interaction and 5 min direct questioning. They also recommend that patients be interviewed jointly by two interviewers, who then complete their ratings independently prior to averaging the results.

The interview relies on the clinical skills of the interviewer to elicit information and to judge the severity of unusual behaviour noted. No criteria are included for rating severity, though these have been suggested by other authors (Wiles *et al.*, 1976; Bigelow and Murphy, 1978). A computer programme is available to facilitate classification (E.C.D.E.U., 1976).

Reliability and validity
Overall and Gorham (1962) report reliability co-efficients of between 0.87 for "Hallucinatory Behaviour" and 0.56 for "Tension". However, these are likely to be overestimates due to the enthusiastic involvement of the authors. Cross centre studies would be more likely to show lower correlations due to the lack of a standardized training programme and also the problems stated below.

Utility
In their review of five psychiatric journals Manchanda *et al.* (1989) found that the BPRS was the most commonly used scale – it was used in 58% of all papers using a rating scale for schizophrenia. Although much used, the BPRS has several drawbacks. At a practical level, it is brief and fairly simple to use but the guidelines are far from adequate, the interviewer/rater needs to be an experienced psychiatrist

(although McGorry *et al.*, 1988, have published a modification for use by nursing staff) and there is no training programme. Furthermore, it is often inconvenient to follow the author's recommendation of having two independent interviewers for every assessment. At a more theoretical level, the "symptom contructs" have no construct validity being developments from factor analysis. The symptoms are not easy to differentiate from one another and bear little relationship to the diagnostic signs and symptoms usually employed in psychiatric practice.

The Present State Examination Change Rating Scale (PSECRS)
(Tress et al., 1987)

The PSECRS was developed to take advantage of the glossary, training programme and structured interview of the Present State Examination (PSE - Wing *et al.*, 1974) (see Chapter 1) but with an increased sensitivity of the rating and a reduction in administration time. The initial interview takes 1 to 1.5 hours to administer, but subsequent interviews take only 10 to 15 min.

The initial interview with the subject follows the usual procedure for a PSE interview (described in Chapter 1). The interviewer, who need not be a psychiatrist but should have some experience with psychiatric patients, will have previously completed a training course in the use of the PSE. The complete, semi-structured interview is administered and scored using the published glossary and guidelines.

Subsequent interviews will be based on those symptoms or signs rated positively at initial interview (i.e. a score of 1 or 2). Each of these symptoms and signs is printed separately on a slip of paper and they are made up into a booklet. Without reference to preceding or subsequent symptoms each symptom is rated on each occasion whether it is unchanged, worse, better or completely remitted compared to the initial interview which should be kept for comparison. The scale runs from 0 - "completely remitted" to 7 - "markedly worsened" with 4 being "unchanged". The questions from the PSE should be used to elicit evidence of change and, at the end of the interview, the general questions should be used to probe for the emergence of any new symptoms. Information from ward staff may also be used as a basis for probes for new symptoms.

Reliability and validity
Tress *et al.* (1987) carried out an inter-rater reliability study using four raters from different backgrounds and experiences following 14 mixed diagnosis patients from admission to an acute ward for 4 weeks. The Intra-class Correlation Coefficient showed inter-rater reliabilities of between 0.75 and 0.99 with the lowest reliabilities being for the behavioural items as was shown by Wing *et al.* (1974). The scale also has good face validity in that symptoms changed with changes in medication and marked improvements in symptoms coincided with discharges.

Utility
Although the PSECRS shows a great deal of promise as a scale having many

advantages and few disadvantages it is very recent and has not been used in any published studies so it is too early to say whether other users will find it as useful as the authors claim.

It is unique in at least one respect in that it measures change and not absolute severity of a symptom. This is a particularly useful attribute when single case studies are being performed and when treatment effects are being monitored over extended periods. Conversely it is probably more difficult to use than absolute scales for group results. It is quick and fairly simple to use, it is based on a thorough training programme, it has a well-defined glossary of symptoms, a semi-structured interview and can be used by anyone who has successfully trained on the PSE.

The Nurses' Observation Scale for Inpatient Evaluation (NOSIE)
(Honigfeld and Klett,1965)

The NOSIE is a behaviour rating scale for chronic schizophrenic inpatients which is administered by ward staff. It is based on continuous observation, and takes 5 to 10 min to score.

The patients are observed during the observation period by nursing staff and rated separately. The scale has 23 items grouped into 7 factors extracted by factor analysis from an original pool of 100 items. Only two of the factors are relevant directly to psychopathology – "manifest psychosis" and "psychotic depression" with three and four behaviours respectively. The behaviours are rated on a five point scale which runs from 0 - "Never", to 4 - "Always". Scores are taken as the mean of the ratings from individual raters.

Reliability and validity
Normative data are presented on 276 chronic schizophrenics. inter-rater reliability was demonstrated by intra-class correlations for pairs of ratings of 0.73 for manifest psychosis and 0.74 for psychotic depression: these are good correlations for behavioural data.

Utility
The NOSIE seems to be a useful scale for rating patients who may be unable to be reached through normal interview techniques such as withdrawn, mute, hostile or hyperactive patients. Continuous observation of behaviour can be rated regularly to provide information about the patient's clinical state. This kind of information is very difficult to rate in the usual interview situation.

The rating itself is quick and simple to use and requires little training and, considering the nature of the ratings, is quite reliable.

The Comprehensive Psychopathological Rating Scale (CPRS)
(Asberg et al.,1978) (see also Chapters 3 and 6)

The CPRS was devised for measuring changes in psychopathology, specifically those which take place in treatment. It takes 45 to 60 min to administer.

The instrument was developed by an interdisciplinary working group to be used either in full or as a pool of terms from which subscales for particular syndromes could be drawn (see schizophrenia subscale). Items were included if relevant to psychiatric illness, liable to change and capable of being detected in a time limited interview. Those items specifically associated with particular syndromes were avoided.

The scale consists of 67 items, 40 based on reported symptoms, 25 on observed behaviour, one global rating and one item relating to the assumed reliability of the interview. Items are scored on a four point Likert scale where 0 = absence of a symptom, 1 = possible deviation for an individual but within normal variation, 2 = symptom which is clearly pathological and 3 = symptom which is pathological to an extreme degree. The use of half steps is recommended to improve sensitivity. The instrument is designed for use by all trained mental health workers with experience of interviewing psychiatric patients. It is suggested that the naturalistic interview should approximate to a clinical psychiatric interview and that it would normally take place at weekly intervals.

Reliability and validity

Jacobsson *et al.* (1978) reported inter-rater reliability in the assessment of schizophrenia using the 39 relevant items from the CPRS. Five doctors rated 14 patients at joint interviews. For all items other than six observed behaviour items, inter-rater correlation coefficients were at least 0.78.

Utility

The CPRS has a number of strengths, which include clear description of items and the focus on items likely to be sensitive to change. As a change measure for schizophrenia it is less specific than other longer rating scales because the symptoms are chosen to provide a broad coverage of psychiatric illnesses. Only a relatively small number of items are clearly relevant and valid for schizophrenia.

Schizophrenia Change Scale (SCS) (also known as the Montgomery Schizophrenia Scale: MSS)
(Montgomery et al., 1978) (see also Chapters 3 and 6)

This rating scale, derived from the longer CPRS, was designed as a brief change rating scale specifically for use in schizophrenia. It takes 10 to 15 min to administer.

This subscale was derived from the CPRS by extracting the 12 items which were most sensitive to change in a group of 36 schizophrenic patients assessed before and after a 4 week course of neuroleptic treatment. Change was defined on the basis of the clinician's global judgement to divide the patients into groups of responders and non-responders. Items included in the scale were those most highly correlated with this measure. As with the longer CPRS, the 12 items are rated on the basis of a flexible clinical interview and scored on a point Likert scale. Higher ratings are made on a composite basis that includes both frequency and severity.

Reliability and Validity
Inter-rater reliability correlations on individual items ranged from 0.54 to 0.99, with the summed reliability in 11 patients rated at various stages of treatment being 0.98. In the test group the scale was found to be more sensitive than the BPRS.

Utility
This subscale has the advantage of being derived from the CPRS, with clearly defined and commonly used items. However, the items are not clearly mutually exclusive and the scale would be of little use with an uncooperative patient. Furthermore, negative symptoms are not represented because they were considered to be unresponsive to change, so this instrument cannot be used as a general symptom scale.

Manchester Scale
(Krawiecka et al., 1977) (see also Chapters 3, 5 and 6)

This is a brief assessment scale designed for monitoring change in patients with a chronic psychosis, where the assessing doctor is familiar with the patient's illness. It takes 10 to 15 min to administer.

The scale consists of eight items which are measured on a five point (0-4) scale. Four items (depression, anxiety, delusions and hallucinations) are based on symptoms reported by the subject. The remaining four items (incoherence or irrelevance of speech, flattened or incongruous affect, poverty of speech or mutism and psychomotor retardation) are based on observation. There are additional items concerning drug side-effects which may be included during drug trials.

The scale is administered as a non-structured interview but with obligatory questions. This information should be used in conjunction with either previous knowledge of the patient or patient's notes, so that ratings are made on the basis of both observed and reported psychopathology. The five points on the scale are: 0 = absence of symptom, 1 = some evidence symptom is present but not pathological, 2 = symptom present just pathological, 3 = moderate symptoms and 4 = severe symptoms. Raters can train themselves with a videotape obtainable from the Department of Psychiatry in Manchester and a short manual for use is appended to the original paper.

Reliability and validity
Inter-rater reliability based on independent assessment of video-taped interviews was reported as high: Kendall coefficient of concordance (w) ranged between 0.64 - 0.87 for reported symptoms and 0.58 - 0.73 for observed items.

Utility
The Manchester scale is brief, simple and has clear guidelines for use. It has been

demonstrated to be sensitive to change (Owens and Johnstone,1980) and as suitable for use where the raters are relatively inexperienced (Manchanda *et al.*, 1986). It includes both negative and positive symptoms and the reliability compares favourably with the BPRS, the most used assessment instrument of this kind (Manchanda *et al.*, 1986). It is a useful instrument for assessing the effectiveness of a treatment intervention where multiple measures are required.

The Global Assessment Scale (GAS)
(Endicott et al., 1976)

This rating scale is designed to place a subject on a single global dimension of mental health. It takes less than five min to administer.

The instrument was designed as an improvement to the Health Rating Scale of Luborsky (1962). It consists of a 100 point scale, where normal individuals score between 71-80. Those scoring above 80 are judged not only to be without illness but to have positive features of mental health. In making a rating an assessor selects the lowest 10 point interval which describes a subject's functioning in the previous week. Within the 10 point interval a subject is placed according to proximity to the intervals immediately above and below. Information for making a rating may come from a range of sources which include direct interview, a reliable informant or case record.

Reliability and validity
Inter-rater reliability was described in five separate sub-studies in the original paper and ranged from 0.61 judged on semi-structured interview transcripts to 0.91 where independent ratings were made of a joint patient interview group. The standard error of rating indicated a 95% chance that a patient will be given a rating within 11.0 points of the true rating. The authors suggest that its validity is supported by correlations with other measures of overall severity, relationships to rehospitalization and sensitivity to change.

Utility
The instrument has the advantages of being simple, rateable from different sources of information and being very quick to complete. It is limited in being merely a global measure and not specific for schizophrenia. It should not be used by itself as a measure of change in schizophrenia but may be useful as an adjunct to other rating scales based on symptom assessment.

Comparative Utility

A number of factors need to be taken into account when selecting a rating scale for clinical use or research purposes.

Comprehensiveness
The available instruments fall into two groups with respect to comprehensiveness of symptoms assessed and administration time. The longer instruments, such as the CPRS, have advantages where a study requires detailed information about the evolution of psychopathology, whilst shorter scales are likely to be more appropriate choices where frequent measures are necessary, such as in monitoring the impact of a therapeutic intervention. Of the available brief scales the Manchester has some advantages in terms of clarity of use, symptom coverage and relevance of items clinically.

Sensitivity to Change
Most of the available instruments are based on absolute measures of psychopathology and do not allow more subtle changes in the intensity, frequency or distress associated with specific symptoms to be assessed. In contrast, the PSE Change Rating Scale, which rates the occurrence and change in specific symptoms found in each patient, would seem better able to take account of such changes and thus offer a more accurate picture of the development and course of a syndrome. Whilst this is clearly an advantage for single case studies, it may prove cumbersome in group studies where it would be necessary to group patients with different levels of symptoms around a common scale before group comparisons could be made.

Specificity
The rating scales vary in the extent to which particular syndromes can be evaluated. Some instruments, such as the GAS and the CPRS, avoid a focus on particular disorders, while others such as the PSE change rating scale may be viewed as covering symptoms likely to occur in schizophrenia with particular thoroughness. Where there is a need to focus on change in particular aspects of a syndrome, e.g. thought disorder, involuntary movements or negative symptoms, scales described elsewhere in the book, e.g. AIMS or SANS would be needed.

Expertise of Assessor
A further consideration lies in the expertise of the personnel necessary for carrying out assessments. Some instruments require specific training programmes (e.g. PSE Change Rating Scale), while others require varying degrees of psychiatric experience (e.g. BPRS and CPRS). Three scales – the nursing version of the BPRS, the NOSIE and the GAS are suitable for use by nursing staff.

Behavioural Signs versus Self-reported Symptoms
It is often apparent that the information gleaned in a formal interview with a patient may be at variance with the reports of staff in daily contact with that patient. Many of the interviews can give reliable ratings of what the patient is prepared to disclose about their mental state, but ratings of behavioural signs tend to be far less reliable because of the short time sample of the interview. In the extreme case of a mute patient the only recourse would be one of the scales based on rating behaviour such

as NOSIE or the nurses' modification of the BPRS. The user of the scales must decide whether a short time sample or continuous observation would be more appropriate to their needs. Where an individual assessment is being made, there is the possibility of using different scales for different problems. However, when group studies are planned the choice of scale may limit the number of patients that can be monitored, as all subjects will need to be compared on the same rating.

References

Asberg, M., Montgomery, S.A., Perris, C., Shalling, D. and Sedvall, G. (1978). The comprehensive psychopathological rating scale. *Acta Psychiatrica Scandinavica, Supplement*, **271**, 5-27.

Bigelow, L. and Murphy, D.L. (1978). Guidelines and anchor points for modified BPRS. NIMH Intramural Research Program, St Elizabeth Hospital, Washington D.C.

Early Clinical Drug Evaluation Unit (1976). "ECDEU" Assessment Manual". D.H.E.W. Rockville, Maryland. *Archives of General Psychiatry, 33*, 766-772.

Endicott, J., Spilzer, R.L., Fless, J.L. and Cohen, J. (1976). The global assessment scale. *Archives of General Psychiatry, 33*, 766-772.

Honigfeld, G. and Klett, C.J. (1965). The nurses' observation scale for inpatient evaluation: A new scale for measuring improvement in chronic schizophrenia. *Journal of Clinical Psychology*, **21**, 65-71.

Jacobsson, L., von Knorring, L., Mattson, B., Perris, C., Edenius, B., Kettner, B., Magnusson, K.E. and Villemoes, P. (1978). The comprehensive psychopathological rating scale – CPRS – in patients with schizophrenic syndromes. Inter-rater reliability and in relation to Marten's S-scale. *Acta Psychiatrica Scandinavica* (suppl). **271**, 39-44.

Krawiecka, M., Goldberg, D. and Vaughan, M. (1977). A standardised psychiatric assessment scale for rating chronic psychiatric patients. *Acta Psychiatrica Scandinavica, 55*, 299 - 308.

Leff, J.P., Tress, K.H. and Edwards, B. (1988). The clinical course of depressive symptoms in schizophrenia. *Schizophrenia Research, 1*, 25-30.

Lorr, M., Jenkins, R.L. and Holsopple, J.Q. (1953). Multidimensional scale for rating psychiatric patients. *Veterans Administration Technical Bulletin, 10*, 507.

Lorr, M., McNair, D.M., Klett, C.J. and Lasky, J.J. (1960). A confirmation of nine postulated psychotic syndromes. *American Psychologist, 15*, 495.

Luborsky, L. (1962). Clinicians' judgement of mental health. *Archives of General Psychiatry, 7*, 407-417.

Manchanda, R., Saupe, R. and Hirsch, S.R. (1986). Comparison between the Brief Psychiatric Rating Scale and the Manchester Scale for the rating of schizophrenic symptoms. *Acta Psychiatrica Scandinavica, 74*, 563-568.

Manchanda, R., Hirsch, S.R. and Barnes, T.R. E. (1989). A review of rating scales for measuring symptom changes in schizophrenia research. *In* "The Instruments of Psychiatric Research". (Ed. C. Thompson), pp. 59-86. John Wiley and Sons, London.

McGorry, P.D., Goodwin, R.J. and Stuart, G.W. (1988). The development of the Brief Psychiatric Rating Scale (nursing modification) – an assessment procedure for the nursing team in clinical and research settings. *Comprehensive Psychiatry, 29*, 575-587.

Montgomery, S.A., Taylor, P. and Montgomery, D. (1978). Development of a schizophrenia scale sensitive to change. Rating Scale. *Neuropharmacology, 17*, 1061-1063.

Overall, J.E. and Gorham, D. R. (1962). The brief psychiatric rating scale. *Psychological Reports*, **10**, 799-812.

Overall, J. and Klett, C. (1972). "Applied Multivariate Analysis". McGraw-Hill, New York.

Owens, D.C.G. and Johnstone, E.C. (1980). The disability of chronic schizophrenia – their nature and factors contributing to their development. *British Journal of Psychiatry*, **136**, 384-395.

Tress, K.H., Belleuis, C., Brownlow, J.M., Livingston, G. and Leff, J.P. (1987). The present state examination change rating scale. *British Journal of Psychiatry*, **150**, 201-207.

Wiles, D., Kolakowska, T., McNeilly, A., Mandelbrote, B. and Gelder, M. (1976). Clinical significance of plasma chlorpromazine level. I. Plasma levels of the drug, some of its metabolites and prolactin during treatment. *Psychological Medicine*, **6**, 407-415.

Wing, J.K., Cooper, J.E. and Sartorius, N. (1974). "The Measurement and Classification of Psychiatric Symptoms". Cambridge University Press, Cambridge.

3. The Assessment of Positive Symptoms

Philippa Garety and Simon Wessely

The term "positive symptoms" was first introduced into medicine in the 19th century by both Reynolds and Hughlings Jackson, albeit with different meanings (Berrios, 1984; Trimble, 1986). In recent years it was reintroduced into psychiatry following the work of Venables and Wing (see Wing, 1989, for review), though it did not become widely used until the work of Crow (1980). It is this latest formulation that remains in use today, and has given rise to the frequent divisions of the symptoms of schizophrenia into positive and negative dimensions.

What are Positive Symptoms?

Most authors agree that positive symptoms refer to the "productive" symptoms of schizophrenia, which consist of delusions, hallucinations and thought disorder. They are called positive or productive because they are regarded as pathological by their presence, rather than by the absence of some aspect of functioning that characterizes negative symptoms. However, there is not absolute agreement as to the precise symptoms that should be regarded as positive. For example, Johnstone *et al.* (1978) include incongruity of affect within the scope of positive symptoms, whilst Andreasen includes several bizarre behaviours within her Scale for the Assessment of Positive Symptoms.

The interest in the positive/negative distinction stems from the suggestion of Crow (1980) that they represent two different disease processes. In his original formulation the positive syndrome was ascribed to an increase in dopamine receptors, whilst the negative resulted from cell loss and cerebral structural change. This theoretical synthesis continues to stimulate much research, and has been supported by several studies in which the clinical correlates of positive and negative features were found to be different (e.g. Owens and Johnstone, 1980: Angrist *et al.*, 1980). However, the division has recently been modified slightly in the light of further research. In particular, Liddle and his colleagues (Liddle, 1987) have shown that schizophrenic symptoms do not readily fall into two groups, but instead can be divided into three categories. The first is labelled psychomotor poverty (i.e. negative symptoms). The second, disorganization, reflects thought disorder and inappropriate affect, whilst the third, reality distortion, contains delusions and hallucinations. It will be seen that Liddle's second and third categories constitute what others call positive symptoms. The organization of this book in fact follows Liddle's division, since although the current chapter is concerned with the assessment of positive symptoms, thought disorder is being covered elsewhere (Cutting).

Problems in Rating Positive Symptoms

Most of the scales that we will be considering do not use a simple dichotomous distinction (as in present/absent). Instead, most use polychotomous scales, for example, ranging from one to five. All imply that going "up the scale" is associated with more serious symptoms. However, there is confusion concerning precisely what this means – since few distinguish between intensity and frequency. Some scales rate on the intensity of the symptom, some on the phenomenology (as in the difference between an over valued idea and a delusion, or a pseudo and true hallucination, e.g. PSE), some on the frequency with which a symptom occurs (e.g. SAPS), some on the severity (e.g. BPRS) and some on a mixture of both (e.g. CPRS). This means that comparing scales is difficult.

A second problem with all the rating scales under consideration is the difficulties of rating thought disorder or incoherence. The methods of rating such disorder are considered elsewhere (Cutting), but may intrude on the rest of the assessment by rendering it impossible to ascertain the presence of any other positive symptoms. All scales thus have a problem with false negatives.

Construct validity   Some researchers, notably Kay and colleagues in New York, Johnstone and her colleagues at Northwick Park, and Andreasen in Iowa, have made efforts to establish construct validity for the assessment of positive symptoms. Construct validity is always a difficult concept in psychiatry, since before claiming such validity it is axiomatic that the reference criterion, whatever that may be, is itself valid. This assumption is often less than perfect (Thorndike and Hagen, 1969) and in general it is better to attempt to multi operationalize measurement than to rely on one scale alone.

However, there is some consensus on three matters concerning positive symptoms, each of which can be used to establish at least some construct validity. These have been listed by Johnstone (1989) as follows:

1   Positive features are characteristic of earlier phases of the illness;
2   Positive symptoms are more drug responsive;
3   Positive features are less stable than negative features.

One method of assessing construct validity is therefore to see how accurate the scale in question is in delineating a group that fulfils these criteria. However, two problems remain. First, it must be conceded that this is rather crude, since each of Johnstone's criteria have been criticized. Second, only recently have attempts been made to assess anything other than the simplest face validity, and thus for most of the scales under consideration such data do not exist.

The Assessment Procedures

Diagnostic instruments include items relating to positive symptoms but they will not be considered in this chapter as they are covered elsewhere (see Chapter 1). General scales designed to cover a broad range of psychopathology will also include a number of items dealing with positive symptoms; these scales will be reviewed here with particular reference to their positive symptoms items. Some scales look more specifically at positive symptoms whilst others focus on a single class of positive symptoms, such as delusions or hallucinations.

Instruments Designed to Record Symptoms in General

Manchester Scale
(Krawiecka et al., 1977) (See Chapter 2 for description, and also Chapters 5 and 6)

In this scale higher ratings are made on a severity dimension: so that for "delusions" a rating of 2 is given for over valued ideas, whilst 3 and 4 are reserved for full delusions. The implication, which is open to question, is that over valued ideas are but a milder form of delusion.

Reliability and validity
Manchanda *et al.* (1986) have demonstrated high reliability (both inter-rater and test-retest) for most items, but especially the positive features. Most of the data on validity come from the studies of Johnstone and colleagues, using the scale divided into positive, negative and non specific sections (Johnstone *et al.*, 1978). They have demonstrated over a 4 year period that negative symptoms as rated by the scale are indeed more stable than positive features. They have also shown in a trial of flupenthixol that the scale successfully discriminated between drug responsive positive symptoms and drug resistant negative symptoms (Johnstone, 1989), confirmed by a trial of propranolol in the treatment of schizophrenia (Manchanda and Hirsch, 1986*b*).

Utility
Manchanda *et al.* (1986) compared the BPRS and the Manchester Scale. Overall, the Manchester Scale performed better, and is probably a better scale for the recording of positive symptoms. Mood disorder is, however, restricted to depression and psychomotor retardation, and thus it would not be suitable for rating populations including manic/schizomanic or schizo-affective subjects, nor when coverage is needed of a wide range of pathology.

Comprehensive Psychopathological Rating Scale (CPRS)
(Asberg et al., 1978) (See Chapter 2 for description, and also Chapter 6)

Reliability and validity
In the Jacobsson *et al.* (1978) study of schizophrenic subjects, high inter-rater reliability was demonstrated for all the positive features. Inter-rater reliability was greater than 0.9 for 14 out of the 16 reported symptoms, and above 0.8 for 16 of the 23 observed items.

Schizophrenia Change Scale (SCS): (also known as the Montgomery Schizophrenia Scale: MSS

(Montgomery et al., 1978) (See Chapter 2 for description, and also Chapter 6)

Reliability and validity

The SCS was derived by a discriminant function analysis of the results of the CPRS in assessing change in symptoms during a 4 week clinical trial of anti-psychotic medication in 36 patients (Montgomery and Montgomery, 1980). It is thus empirically chosen on the basis of symptoms that respond to medication rather than from any theoretical perspective. Its usefulness in assessing positive symptoms is thus based on the observation that such symptoms preferentially respond to medication.

Utility

One limitation in the assessment of positive symptoms is that coverage of hallucinations is restricted to commenting voices only: this is because the other CPRS symptoms were not found empirically to be of use in assessing change. Also, some of the subscales are rather overlapping – what is the precise difference between delusional mood and perplexity, for example ?

It should be noted that although listed as a general symptom scale the SCS has no coverage of negative symptoms and so should be considered as for the rating of positive symptoms only.

Brief Psychiatric Rating Scale (BPRS)

(Overall and Gorham, 1962) (See Chapter 2 for description)

Utility

Manchanda and Hirsch (1986a) have pointed out that the subjective nature of the ratings of severity mean that it is difficult to compare results between centres. Reliability is also adversely affected by the absence of a standard time period for rating.

The scale was constructed for use in treatment studies of general psychiatric disorders, and was derived from factor analysis of even longer scales than the final version (Overall, 1974). Since it was designed for general use, not many of the items are specific to schizophrenia, and only four or perhaps five, could even with the widest possible interpretation, be considered to be recording positive features (conceptual disorganization, hallucinatory behaviour, unusual thought content, suspiciousness and grandiosity). A particular problem is the assessment of delusions; these must be unusual to be recorded, but could then be rated under both "unusual thought content" and "suspiciousness". Thus it lacks even reasonable face validity for any study of the positive/negative distinction.

Instruments Designed To Record Positive Symptoms

The Positive and Negative Syndrome Scale (PANSS)
(Kay et al., 1988 and 1989) (see also Chapter 5)

The PANSS rates positive and negative features of schizophrenia for both basic and treatment studies. There is an interview with the patient, taking 30-40 min, and this information is supplemented by details obtained from staff/relatives, etc.

The scale comprises 30 items, of which seven are labelled positive and seven negative items: the remaining 16 items constitute a general psychopathology scale. The positive items are delusions, conceptual disorganization, hallucinatory behaviour, excitement, grandiosity, suspiciousness/persecution and hostility. Each item is scored 1 to 7, in which 1 is absent.

Operational criteria are provided for each item, listed in a Rating Manual (obtainable from the author (see page vii)). Ratings are not made simply on the result of the interview, but should also be based on observations by staff and relatives. Higher ratings are made on a composite basis, mainly frequency but also behavioural disruption. The rating period is usually the past week, but this can be altered.

The number of positive and negative items is deliberately balanced, so that the difference between the two is a composite scale which according to the authors, "expresses the extent of predominance of one syndrome over the other".

Reliability and validity
Kay and colleagues have accumulated substantial reliability data from a study of 101 chronic schizophrenics. Inter-rater and split-half reliability data, as well as coefficient alpha (Cronbach's alpha), are listed by Kay *et al.* (1987, 1989), and all are very acceptable. Test-retest reliability was calculated over a 3 to 6 month period using a subsample of treatment non responders (to minimize, but not eliminate, subject variability) and the Pearson's correlation coefficient was 0.80 for the positive items.

In an effort to improve content validity the PANSS included items covering several different areas of functioning, namely, cognitive, affective, social and communicative. The items were adapted from two previous scales, the Psychopathology Rating Scale originating from the same group, and the BPRS.

Concurrent validity was established by comparison with the Andreasen scales mentioned in the next section – the Pearson correlation coefficient between the two was 0.77 for the positive scales. Of course, it is still possible that both measures are flawed. Negative correlation between the two scales (positive and negative) is also proposed as evidence for construct validity. Criterion validity is suggested by a study using independent clinical, genetic and psychometric measures. A different pattern of associations was observed for each of the two scales. This was also replicated in two subsequent samples. Finally, a further criterion validity (in this case predictive validity) was suggested by a trial of L-DOPA in which significant improvements were noted on the negative, but not the positive, scales, which was taken as further evidence of construct validity.

Utility

Kay *et al.* have gone to considerable trouble to create scales that are consistent with the underlying positive/negative construct. They also have attempted to include unambiguous items which they regard as primary (thus they exclude preoccupation, as that may be secondary to either hallucinations or "arousal disorder"). The authors have performed an impressive number of validation studies, but as yet the Scale has not been used outside their centre.

Scale for the Assessment of Positive Symptoms (SAPS)
(Andreasen, 1984)

The SAPS rates positive symptoms in schizophrenia and is intended to be used in conjunction with the Scale for the Assessment of Negative Symptoms, and the Comprehensive Assessment of Symptoms and History (CASH). It is administered as a general clinical interview, followed by standardized questions, but ratings should also include information from other sources, such as staff and case notes. Normally, the time period covered is the previous month, but it can be used for other periods, e.g. last week, etc.

The great strength of this scale is the detailed clinical definitions given of a large number of symptoms to be rated independently. Thus hallucinations are rated under six items (auditory, voices commenting, voices conversing, somatic or tactile, olfactory and finally visual hallucinations). Items are scored 0 to 5. There is some inconsistency in scaling – for hallucinations increasing scores are indicated by frequency, with a separate item for severity. However, the rating of delusions is a mixture of conviction, severity and preoccupation, and also includes a measure of delusional action (for many delusional items the maximal rating can only be given if the subject acts on the abnormal belief). This may give rise to some problems, since not only may delusional behaviour be a different construct, it will also influence ratings under bizarre behaviour. Furthermore, conviction and preoccupation do not necessarily covary (Garety and Hemsley, 1987; Brett-Jones *et al.*, 1987). The Scale also covers positive thought disorder, such as derailment, incoherence and pressure, and provides excellent detailed descriptions for each item.

Reliability and validity

Very little has been published as yet on the SAPS. It has been used in one phenomenological study (Kulhara *et al.*, 1986), but although inter-rater reliability data were made available for the SANS, none was presented for the SAPS. So far it appears that the only published data derive from an Italian version of the SAPS (Moscarelli *et al.*, 1987). Twenty-four schizophrenics were rated by two psychiatrists using both the SAPS and the SANS. As judged by Cronbach's alpha, the internal reliability of the four sections (hallucinations, delusions, bizarre behaviour and formal thought disorder) of the SAPS is good. Furthermore, weighted kappas for nearly all the items were very satisfactory, mostly between 0.7 and 1.00 the only exception being delusions of jealousy. One extra piece of information was that although no specific training is required for the SAPS, when the same procedure was carried out by medical students "experienced in psychiatry" very poor results, which were not quoted, were obtained. The authors also quoted two other unpublished studies of the SAPS from Spain and Japan as giving acceptable reliabilities. Since then Andreason has summarized experience with both the SAPS and re SANS in a useful chapter (Andreasen, 1990). Overall, inter-rater reliability is satisfactory for most items on the SAPS, although, as one might predict, values are generally higher for hallucinations and delusions than bizarre behaviour and thought disorder. Andreasen (1990) also presents data on internal consistency, which suggested that positive symptoms in general were less internally cohesive than negative ones.

Instruments Designed to Record Specific Positive Symptoms

Delusions

Personal Questionnaire Assessments of Conviction and Preoccupation
(Garety, 1985; Brett-Jones et al., 1987)

This technique assesses conviction and pre-occupation with delusional beliefs and is sensitive to small changes over repeated measures. The questionnaire, which is tailored to the individual patient and his/her delusions, takes approximately 10 min to construct. Thereafter a single questionnaire is normally administered in 5 min.

Shapiro's Personal Questionnaire (PQ) is a technique for measuring psychological changes specific to individual psychiatric patients (Shapiro, 1961). A later modification of Phillips (1977) is employed. To construct a PQ written statements are chosen by the subject to represent different levels of symptom intensity. The statements are written on separate cards and are ranked by the subject. In the administration of the questionnaire the cards are presented to the subject in random order, one at a time. For each card the subject must make a choice as to whether, at the time of presentation, the symptom is of greater or lesser intensity than is stated on the card. The score on each occasion is given by the number of cards to which the subject replies that the symptom intensity is greater than that shown on the card. The symptom chosen may differ for each subject, as may the statements of intensity. The questionnaire thus aims only to give an ordinal scale which allows for comparisons within a subject across time, but not between subjects.

The PQ technique differs from unstructured self-report in that it provides for a scaling of a symptom with a check on internal consistency, and it differs from other questionnaire forms in that it is devised for each individual, using that person's words to describe their beliefs, experiences or feelings. Although PQ assessments of conviction and preoccupation are described here, the PQ has also been used to assess other relevant aspects of the subject's mental state such as distress about the delusional belief.

Conviction

Subjects are asked to choose their own wording for five statements of intensity of conviction; an example of such a set might be:

I doubt that; I have few doubts that; I feel fairly sure that; I believe very strongly that; I know/I am absolutely certain that.

Preoccupation

Subjects again choose their own wording to represent different degrees of preoccupation with the target belief; for example:

I think about these things not at all; ....occasionally; ....some of the time;....most of the time ....absolutely all the time.

(Note that with a PQ, a 6 point ordinal scale results from a 5 statement scaling. This is because the points of the ordinal scale lie in between or outside the statements used.)

Although the PQ is an essentially idiographic technique it has been employed to measure longitudinal change in intensity of conviction and level of preoccupation in studies investigating series of single cases: Garety, 1985 (8 subjects), Brett-Jones *et al.,* 1987 (nine cases); Grossman, 1989 (nine cases) and Chadwick and Lowe, 1990 (six cases).

Reliability and validity

Inconsistency of responses can be detected by the tester, and corrected immediately. Errors resulting from inattention or failure to understand the task are therefore minimized. Test-retest reliability, within a session, was calculated by Brett-Jones *et al.* on 34 interviews and weighted kappas of 0.89 for conviction and of 0.63 for preoccupation (both $p < 0.002$) were obtained.

Chadwick and Lowe (1990), following Hole *et al.* (1979) asked subjects for percentage ratings of conviction, and reported that these subjective ratings correlated very highly ($r = 0.99$) with PQ scores. However, these ratings were taken directly after the PQ measures and so may not have been independent.

Utility

PQ measures are most useful for the monitoring of different aspects of delusional beliefs over time. They may be used to assess treatment effects or to monitor the rate of change in dimensions of belief. As a research tool the technique is most useful in single case designs.

The PSE (see Chapter 1) also assesses conviction in delusional belief, but this is only categorized into "full" or "partial" conviction, so changes within the range of "partial" cannot be detected by this instrument.

Reaction of Hypothetical Contradiction and Accommodation
(Brett-Jones et al., 1987)

This technique assesses the potential or actual impact of information incompatible with the subject's delusion on the belief. Each measure takes less than 5 min.

Reaction to hypothetical contradiction (RTHC) is a method of categorizing a subject's potential for accommodating evidence contradictory to the belief. Subjects are presented with a hypothetical but concrete and plausible piece of evidence contradictory to the belief, and asked how this would affect their belief. Replies are assigned to one of four categories.

Accommodation assesses the awareness of the subject of actual occurrences contradictory to the belief. Subjects are asked if anything has happened to alter their belief in any way over the past week and replies are assigned to one of five categories.

Reliability and validity
Brett-Jones *et al.* report inter-rater reliabilities, on a sample of 27 interviews, using weighted kappas, of 0.74 ($p < 0.002$) for RTHC and of 0.75 ($p < 0.002$) for accommodation.

Utility
Brett-Jones *et al.* found that those subjects who were willing to consider a reduction in conviction in the face of hypothetical contradictory evidence were more likely to show subsequently a rejection of their beliefs. Chadwick and Lowe (1990) found a similar pattern in a treatment study of chronically deluded patients. They also found that while no subject reported a single instance of accommodation in the baseline period, after the introduction of cognitive behavioural therapy, subjects reported instances of disconfirmation. The value of these measures is currently a matter largely of thoretical interest, although they may also have therapeutic implications.

Characteristics of Delusions Rating Scale
(Garety and Hemsley, 1987)

This scale assesses the subjective characteristics of delusions, using a visual analogue technique. It is suitable for most deluded patients, and is administered in about 20 min.

The scale incorporates a total of 11 belief characteristics, which are capable of being assessed by the individual holding the belief, rather than by an observer. These are represented on paper as a line which has at each end a brief description of the opposite extremes of the dimension; e.g. for conviction the end-points of the line are "believe absolutely" and "believe not at all". The other characteristics are: preoccupation, interference (identifiable influence on behaviour), resistance, dismissibility, absurdity, worry, unhappiness, reassurance seeking, self-evidentness and pervasiveness.

The belief to be rated is first elicited by the interviewer, and the wording agreed with the subject. The rating scale is then administered with the interviewer explaining and clarifying each item and the subject invited to make a mark with a pencil at any point along the line to indicate the degree to which the characteristic described represented her/his experience. The scale is scored using a template with ten equal divisions.

Reliability and validity
No test-retest reliability is reported. More recently, the same technique (although measuring different variables) has been used on nine deluded subjects each seen on 10 occasions (90 interviews) (Grossman, 1989). Test-retest reliabilities were high: Cronbach's alpha coefficient, $x = 0.82$, (S.D. 0.21).

Correlations between variables measuring related constructs were positive, and a principal components analysis yielded four components.

Utility
A visual analogue scale is rapidly administered and easily understood by even floridly deluded subjects. The reliability and validity of the technique with this population requires further investigation. It has the advantage of assessing a variety of features of a delusion. Its sensitivity to change is unknown.

Personal Ideation Inventory (PII)
(Rattenbury et al., 1984)

The Personal Ideation Inventory (PII) is a semi-structured interview designed for use in research to focus on major dimensions of delusional ideation. It consists of 71 items that assess various aspects of the content of a delusion, including its relation to pre-morbid concerns and the extent of a patient's conviction, commitment, and perspective to his/her central delusion. Conviction refers to how strongly the patient believes his/her delusional ideas are real or true, whilst Commitment refers to the immediacy of the belief, or how impelling or important it feels to the patient. This latter measure is based on cognitive signs, preoccupation with and dismissibility of the delusion, and behavioural signs, influence on daily activities. The final score for this dimension is a composite score. Perspective refers to the patient's view about whether others will regard his/her ideas as strange or implausible. The interviewer assigns scores to the subject's response, based on predetermined categories. Questions refer to both the present and to the time at which the delusion was at its height.

Reliability and validity
Harrow et al. (1988) report inter-rater reliability coefficients from 14 taped interviews for belief conviction, perspective and emotional commitment of 0.82, 0.81 and 0.77 respectively.

Correlation coefficients are, however, no longer regarded as the first choice statistic for assessing inter-rater reliabilities; kappas are generally recommended.

A problem with the PII is the focus on three "dimensions" of delusions, in which responses to a number of questions are summed to generate a final score. "Emotional commitment" combines responses about preoccupation, dismissibility and behaviour. There is no explicit justification for this. Correlations between dimensions are reported: conviction correlates positively with perspective ($r = 0.58$) and with commitment ($r = 0.51$); the latter two dimensions are non-significantly correlated at 0.21.

Utility
The PII is a research tool. It brings together an existing measure, content ratings from the SADS, with questions about the development of the delusion, and the dimensions. However, there may be some doubt as to the validity of emotional commitment as a unitary dimension, since belief and behaviour may not be highly correlated. The value of assessing perspective in such detail is at present largely theoretical.

Scales for Rating Psychotic and Psychotic-like Experiences as Continua
(Chapman and Chapman, 1980)

This scale is a modification of parts of the Schedule for Affective Disorders and Schizophrenia-Lifetime version (SADS-L), (Spitzer and Endicott, 1977), an interview commonly used for diagnosing a variety of psychiatric disorders. The modifications consist of the addition of questions about attenuated forms of the same symptoms (including delusions and hallucinations) that are used in SADS-L to diagnose psychosis. Scores are assigned between 1 and 11 on judgements of increasing deviancy. Details are given in the paper.

Reliability and validity
Reliability is reported in Chapman and Chapman, (1980). A coefficient alpha of 0.94 was obtained from six expert judges on the deviancy ratings. Sixty-nine interview excerpts (one subject) were rated by two judges at a correlation of 0.78. Subjects who scored highly on an assessment of magical ideation were identified as high scorers on this scale (see below).

Magical Ideation Scale (MIS)
(Eckblad and Chapman, 1983)

The MIS, for use with normals, is a 30 item scale designed to measure belief in forms of causation that by conventional standards are invalid (within a North American culture), such as thought transmission, psychokinetic effects, precognition, and the transfer of psychic energies between people. Most of the items inquire about the subject's interpretation of his or her own personal experiences rather than belief in the theoretical possibility of magical forms of causation. The scale is intended to identify young adults who may be psychosis prone.

The MIS is a self-administered scale, each item to be endorsed as true or false, and can be completed in 5 min.

Reliability and validity

The MIS was standardized on 1512 college students, with mean scores of 8.56 (S.D. 5.24) for men and of 9.69 (S.D. 5.93) for women. The Coefficient alpha is > 0.80. It correlates 0.32 with the Eysenck Psychoticism Scale and 0.68 (Men) and 0.71 (Women) with the Perceptual Aberration Scale of Chapman *et al.* (1976).

Subjects interviewed on the modified SADS-L (as described above) who scored high on the MIS showed more psychotic-like and schizotypal symptoms than control subjects.

Utility

Both of these scales are of interest to researchers concerned with studies of high risk for psychosis, and for studying aberrant beliefs. Note: the Scales for rating psychotic and psychotic-like experiences as continua (Chapman and Chapman, 1980), also include items relevant to the study of hallucinations.

Dimensions of Delusional Experience Scale (DDES)
(Kendler et al., 1983)

This scale was developed to measure five postulated dimensions of delusional experience, and to investigate their relative independence.

The dimensions are conviction, extension (the degree to which the delusional belief involves different areas of the patient's life), bizarreness, disorganization and pressure (preoccupation and concern). The scale is administered as a semistructured interview lasting 45 min. Ratings are made by the interviewer; extension and disorganization are measured on a 3 point ordinal scale, conviction on a 4 point ordinal scale and bizarreness and pressure on a 5 point ordinal scale.

Reliability and validity

Reliability of the ratings was assessed by interviewing 23 subjects in the presence of a second rater. Weighted kappas of between 0.80 (for conviction) and 0.30 (for bizarreness) were obtained (all p <0.05). The intercorrelations between different dimensions were uniformly low, supporting the hypothesis of delusions as multi-dimensional.

Utility

This is an observer-rated scale, achieving adequate (except for bizarreness) but not high, inter-rater reliabilities on a number of dimensions. Little other information is presented. The authors rightly argue for the assessment of other aspects of delusions besides conviction. It is, however, possible to use other scales/techniques, about which more information is available, for this.

Hallucinations

The Launay-Slade Hallucination Scale (LSHS)
(Launay and Slade, 1981)

This is a 12 item questionnaire to measure hallucinatory predisposition in normals. It includes both pathological items and items representing sub-clinical forms of hallucinatory experience, such as vivid thoughts and daydreams. The subject is required to endorse each item as true or false. The form can be completed in less than 5 min.

Reliability and validity
The scale was first tested with three groups, normals (prison psychologists), prisoners and psychiatric patients. Normals ($n = 54$) scored 1.7 (S.D. 1.66), prisoners ($n = 200$) 5.08 (S.D. 2.87) and hallucinating patients ($n = 42$) 7.75 (S.D. 2.44). The test-retest reliability of the scale was studied by Bentall and Slade (1985) using a modified version. Subjects were 150 male undergraduate students, and were given two slightly different versions of the scale with an inter-test interval of between 2 days and 3 weeks. The Pearson product-moment correlation coefficient was 0.84 ($p < 0.0001$). Young *et al.* (1987) report a study relevant to the validity of the scale.

Subjects scoring high on the LSHS were significantly more likely to hear suggested sounds and to see suggested objects than low scorers ($p < 0.05$).

Utility
This scale is primarily a research tool, assisting in the study of hallucination-like experiences and hallucination-proneness in the normal population.

The Reality Characteristics of Hallucinations
(Aggernaes, 1972)

Aggernaes describes a structured interview to assess seven "reality characteristics" of hallucinations. These include assessing whether the experience has the quality of perception or of imagination, or of "publicness" versus "privateness". The interview is suitable for use with hallucinating patients, with both chronic and acute psychoses, and has been conducted with LSD drug abusers. Aggernaes specifies probe questions to clarify responses, and argues against standardization of the interview, instead suggesting the use of supplementary questions to double-check responses. Where a patient changes his or her response as a result, a "doubtful" classification is made.

Reliability and validity
Aggernaes and his colleagues report studies with 41 hallucinating schizophrenics, 29 LSD drug abusers, and of "normal" experiences of 15 non-psychotic patients (see also Slade and Bentall, 1988, for details). Aggernaes and Byeborg (1972) report on the test-retest and inter-rater reliability of the interview, with 35 hallucinating patients. 88% agreement was reported on re-interviews with a 1-2 month interval, and 85% for inter-rater reliability, although the authors comment on the limitations of percentage agreement as a measure. Aggernaes and Byeborg (1972) also report a study in which hallucinated patients are asked to imagine an object and to describe the reality characteristics of the experience. Subjects' responses clearly demonstrated a capacity to experience such an image as non-existent, and thus affords the interview some divergent validation.

Utility
The interview is potentially a very valuable research tool in that it takes detailed information about the experienced characteristics of hallucinations, conceptualized within a theoretical framework. The reliability warrants further study.

Perceptual Characteristics of Auditory Hallucinations
(Alpert and Silvers, 1970)

This is a structured interview to investigate the sensory, perceptual and cognitive characteristics of hallucinations.

A questionnaire requiring only yes/no answers is completed by the interviewer on the basis of a 2-3 hour interview. The questionnaire is not given in full by Alpert and Silvers (1970); only eight questions are reported, concerning frequency, localization of source, change in frequency with arousal, isolation or light, and verbal/nonverbal content.

Reliability and validity
Alpert and Silvers report on responses from 45 schizophrenics and 18 patients with alcoholic hallucinosis but no reliability data are reported. Differences between the groups of hallucinators offer some divergent validation.

Utility
The utility of this potential measure is strictly limited by the limited details given of the questionnaire items, but some interesting questions are listed.

Auditory Hallucinations Record Form
(Slade, 1972)

The Record Form aims to identify the factors which precipitate the experience of auditory hallucinations in a given patient. The patient records on the form, at pre-determined times, the presence/absence of "voices", their intensity, a series of subjectively assessed environmental variables (e.g. noise, people, activity), mood state and 15 semantic differential scales to assess the "quality" of the "voices". The patient is asked to complete the form three times a day for a period of a few weeks. The data from the environmental and mood variables are then contrasted for the occasions on which the voices are present/absent.

Reliability and validity
No standardization, reliability or validity data are reported.

Utility
The Record Form is designed for clinical use within a single case framework. It may lead to hypotheses regarding the precipitating factors of hallucinations, e.g. increased arousal, and treatment implications. Slade (1972 and 1973) reports on two such cases.

Scales for Rating Psychotic and Psychotic-like Experiences as Continua
(Chapman and Chapman, 1980)

This scale, which includes measures of hallucinations as well as delusions, has been described earlier (p. 33)

Measures of Characteristics of Hallucinations

A number of individual treatment studies have reported measures of aspects of hallucinations (see Slade and Bentall, 1988, for comprehensive list of references), which include measures of frequency, intensity, duration, clarity, volume and intrusivenss. These are not standardized measures, but are potentially useful for single case treatment studies.

Conclusions

General Scales
Scales for the assessment of positive symptoms of schizophrenia are used for two purposes. The first is for treatment trials, in which an easily administered scale sensitive to change is required. The second is for more basic research into the positive/negative distinction, and its underlying validity. Our opinion is that the Manchester Scale probably represents the best instrument for the former, although the SCS is still acceptable. For more fundamental research the choice is between the SAPS and the PANSS. Both are well constructed, and whilst the PANSS has more published reliability data, the SAPS is particularly strong on phenomenologically precise definitions. In practice it is probable that there is little to choose between the two, and that both are acceptable for detailed studies.

Specific Scales

Many of the specific procedures treat delusions as a multi-dimensional phenomenon, a view for which empirical support is strong. Which are the important dimensions is, however, less clear. Garety and Hemsley (1987) describe 11 characteristics, and from them derive four principal components; Kendler *et al.* (1983) derive two factors from five variables; Rattenbury *et al.* (1984) take as their starting point three dimensions. All consider belief-conviction as an important (perhaps the most important) dimension; preoccupation achieves wide recognition; behaviour related to the belief is also of interest, but clearly the measures presented here are as yet unrefined attempts at assessment.

Other dimensions favoured by some, are distress, perspective/insight and systematization. Very little work has yet been done to relate these dimensions to outcome, or to other aspects of the subjects' psychopathology or demographics.

There are surprisingly few scales of proven reliability and validity which provide detailed information about hallucinations. The relationships between the different variables, such as frequency, intensity, dismissibility, and localization have likewise been subject to little systematic study. At present the clinician and researcher are advised to assess a number of the relevant variables.

Acknowledgements

SW is supported by the Wellcome Trust

References

Aggernaes, A. (1972). The experienced reality of hallucinations and other psychological phenomena. *Acta Psychiatrica Scandinavica,* **48**, 220-238.

Aggernaes, A. and Byeborg, O. (1972). The reliability of different aspects of the experienced reality of hallucinations in clear states of consciousness. *Acta Psychiatrica Scandinavica,* **48**, 239-252.

Alpert, M. and Silvers, K.N. (1970). Perceptual characteristics distinguishing auditory hallucinations in schizophrenia and acute alcoholic psychosis. *American Journal of Psychiatry,* **127**, 298-302.

Andreasen, N. (1984). "Scale for the Assessment of Positive Symptoms. (SAPS)". Department of Psychiatry, Iowa City.

Andreasen, N. (1990). Methods for assessing positive and negative symptoms. *In* "Schizophrenia: Positive and Negative Symptoms and Syndromes. Modern Problems in Pharmacopsychiatry". (Ed. N. Andreasen). pp. 73-85. Karger, Basel.

Angrist, B., Rotrosen, J. and Gershon, S. (1980). Differential effects of amphetamine and neuroleptics on negative versus positive symptoms in schizophrenia. *Psychopharmacologia,* **72**, 17-19.

Asberg, M., Montgomery, S., Perris, C., Schalling, D. and Sedvall, G. (1978), The comprehensive psychopathological rating scale. *Acta Psychiatrica Scandinavica,* Suppl **277**, 5-27.

Bentall, R.P., Slade, P.D. (1985). Reliability of a scale measuring disposition towards hallucination: a brief report. *Personality and Individual Differences,* **4**, 527-529.

Berrios, G. (1984). Positive and negative symptoms and Jackson: a conceptual history. *Archives of General Psychiatry, 42*, 95-97.

Brett-Jones, J., Garety, P. and Hemsley, D. (1987). Measuring delusional experiences: a method and its application. *British Journal of Clinical Psychology, 26*, 257-265.

Chadwick, P. and Lowe, C. (in press). The modification of delusional beliefs. *Journal of Consulting and Clinical Psychology.*

Chapman, L.J. and Chapman, J.P. (1980). Scales for rating psychotic and psychotic like experiences as continua. *Schizophrenia Bulletin, 6*, 476-489.

Chapman, L.J., Chapman, J.P. and Raulin, M.L. (1978). Body-image aberration in schizophrenia. *Journal of Abnormal Psychology, 87*, 399-407.

Crow, T. (1980). Molecular pathology of schizophrenia: more than one dimension of pathology? *British Medical Journal, 280*, 66-68.

Eckblad, M. and Chapman, L.J. (1983). Magical ideation as an indicator of schizotypy. *Journal of Consulting and Clinical Psychology, 51*, 215-225.

Garety, P.A. (1985). Delusions: Problems in definition and measurement. *British Journal of Medical Psychology, 58*, 25-34.

Garety, P.A. and Hemsley, D.R. (1987). Characteristics of delusional experience. *European Archives of Psychiatry and Neurological Science, 266*, 294-298.

Grossman A. (1989). Single case longitudinal studies investigating the relationship between delusional beliefs and mood state. Unpublished MSc thesis, Institute of Psychiatry, University of London.

Harrow, M., Rattenbury, F. and Stoll, F. (1988). Schizophrenic delusions: an analysis of their persistence, of related premorbid ideas and of three major dimensions. Ch.9. *In* "Delusional Beliefs". (Eds T.E. Oltmanns and B.A. Maher). Wiley, New York.

Hole, R.W., Rush, A.J. and Beck, A.T. (1979). A cognitive investigation of schizophrenic delusions. *Psychiatry, 42*, 312-319.

Hyde, C. (1989). The Manchester Scale: A Standardised Psychiatric Assessment for Rating Chronic Psychotic Patients. *British Journal of Psychiatry, 155*, Suppl 7, 45-47.

Jacobsson, L., Von Knorring, L., Mattsson, B., Perris, C., Edenius, B., Kettner, B., Magnusson, K. and Villemos, P. (1978). The comprehensive psychopathological rating scale – CPRS – in patients with schizophrenia. *Acta Psychiatrica Scandinavica, 271*, 39-44.

Johnstone, E., Crow, T., Frith, C., Carney, M. and Price, J. (1978). Mechanism of the antipsychotic effect in the treatment of acute schizophrenia. *Lancet, i*, 848-851.

Johnstone, E. (1989). The assessment of positive and negative features in schizophrenia. *British Journal of Psychiatry, 155*, Suppl 7, 41-44.

Kay, S., Fiszbein, A. and L. Opler, (1987). The positive and negative syndrome scale (PANSS) for schizophrenia. *Schizophrenia Bulletin, 13*, 261-275.

Kay, S., Opler, L. and Lindenmayer, J.P. (1988). Reliability and validity of the Positive and Negative Syndrome Scale for schizophrenics. *Psychiatry Research, 23*, 99-110.

Kay, S., Opler, L. and Lindenmayer, J-P. (1989). The Positive and Negative Syndrome Scale (PANSS): Rationale and Standardisation. *British Journal of Psychiatry, 155*, Suppl 7, 59-65.

Kendler, K.S., Glazer, W.M. and Morgenstern, H. (1983). Dimensions of delusional experience. *American Journal of Psychiatry, 140*, 59-65.

Krawiecka, M., Goldberg, D. and Vaughan, M. (1977). A standardised psychiatric assessment scale for rating chronic psychotic patients. *Acta Psychiatrica Scandinavica, 55*, 299-308.

Kulhara, P., Kota, S. and Joseph, S. (1986). Positive and negative subtypes of schizophrenia: A study from India. *Acta Psychiatrica Scandinavica,* **74**, 353-359.

Launay, G. and Slade, P.D. (1981). The measurement of hallucinatory predisposition in male and female prisoners. *Personality and Individual Differences,* **2**, 221-234.

Liddle, P. (1987). The symptoms of chronic schizophrenia: a re-examination of the positive-negative dichodomy. *British Journal of Psychiatry,* **151**, 145-151.

Manchanda, R. and Hirsch, S. (1986*a*). Rating scales for clinical studies in schizophrenia. *In* "The Pharmacology and Treatment of Schizophrenia". (Eds P. Bradley and S. Hirsch), pp. 234-262. Oxford University Press.

Manchanda, R. and Hirsch, S. (1986*b*). Does propranolol have an antipsychotic effect: A placebo controlled study in acute schizophrenia. *British Journal of Psychiatry,* **148**, 701-707.

Manchanda, R., Saupe, R. and Hirsch, S. (1986). Comparison between the brief psychiatric rating scale and the Manchester scale for the rating of schizophrenia symptomatology. *Acta Psychiatrica Scandinavica,* **74**, 563-568.

Manchanda, R., Hirsch, S. and Barnes, T. (1989). A review of rating scales for measuring symptom changes in schizophrenia research. *In* "The Instruments of Psychiatric Research". (Ed. C. Thompson). John Wiley, Chichester.

Montgomery, S. and Montgomery, D. (1980). Measurement of change in psychiatric illness: new obsessional, schizophrenia and depression scales. *Postgraduate Medical Journal,* **50**, Suppl 1, 50-52.

Montgomery, S., Taylor, P. and Montgomery, D. (1978). Development of a schizophrenia scale sensitive to change. *Neuropharmacology,* **17**, 1061-1063.

Moscarelli, M., Maffei, C., Cesana, B. *et al.* (1987). An international perspective on assessment of negative and positive symptoms in schizophrenia. *American Journal of Psychiatry,* **144**, 1595-1598.

Overall, J. (1974). The brief psychiatric rating scale in psychopharmacology research. *In* "Psychological Measures in Psychopharmacology. Modern Problems in Psychiatry". Vol. 7. (Ed. P. Pichot), pp. 67-78. Karger, Basel.

Overall, J. and Gorham, D. (1962). The brief psychiatric rating scale. *Psychological Reports,* **10**, 799-812.

Owens, D. and Johnstone, E. (1980). The disabilities of chronic schizophrenia: their nature and the factors contributing to their development. *British Journal of Psychiatry,* **136**, 384-396.

Phillips, J.P.N. (1977). Generalized personal questionnaire techniques Ch. *In* "The Measurement of Intrapersonal Space by Grid Techniques". Vol. II (Ed. P. Slater). Wiley, London.

Rattenbury, F.R., Harrow, M., Stoll, F.J. and Kettering, R.L. (1984). "The Personal Ideation Inventory: An interview for assessing major dimensions of delusional thinking". Microfiche Publications, New York.

Shapiro, M.B. (1961). A method of measuring psychological disorders specific to the individual psychiatric patient. *British Journal of Medical Psychology,* **34**, 151-155.

Slade, P.D. (1972). The effects of systematic desensitization on auditory hallucinations. *Behavioural Research and Therapy,* **10**, 85-91.

Slade, P.D. (1973). The psychological investigation and treatment of auditory hallucinations: a second case report. *British Journal of Medical Psychology,* **46**, 293.

Slade, P.D. and Bentall, R.P. (1988). "Sensory Deception: A Scientific analysis of hallucination". Croom Helm, London.

Spitzer, R.L. and Endicott, J. (1977). "Schedule for Affective Disorders and Schizophrenia

– Lifetime Version (SADS-L)". New York State Psychiatric Institute, New York.

Thorndike, R. and Hagen, E. (1969). "Measurement and Evaluation in Psychology and Education". (3rd edn.). John Wiley, New York.

Trimble, M. (1986). Positive and negative symptoms in psychiatry. *British Journal of Psychiatry*, **148**, 587-589.

Wing, J. (1989). The concept of negative symptoms. *British Journal of Psychiatry,* **155**, Suppl. 7, 10-14.

Young, H.F., Bentall, R.P., Slade, P.D. and Dewey, M.E. (1987). The role of brief instructions and suggestibility in the elicitation of auditory and visual hallucinations in normal and psychiatric subjects. *Journal of Nervous and Mental Diseases*, **175**, 41-48.

4. The Assessment of Thought Disorder

John Cutting

Thought disorder is notoriously difficult to assess. This is partly because it is a heterogeneous entity and partly because, in most instances of psychosis, it shows itself in only subtle ways.

What thought disorder represents has taxed the ingenuity of all those who have studied it, from Kraepelin and Bleuler to the present day. In this book we are not concerned with the nature of psychotic phenomena, only with current ways of measuring them. For a discussion of the nature of thought disorder see Cutting (1990).

Measures of thought disorder fall into two types. First, there are those which purport to reflect some global abnormality. Then there are those which attempt to detect a more specific abnormality. The former are chiefly clinical and diagnostic assessment procedures. The latter are chiefly psychological tests.

General Assessment Procedures

Thought, Language and Communication Scale (TLC Scale)
(Andreasen, 1979)

This is a comprehensive assessment of thought disorder for use with psychotic subjects (manics, depressives, schizophrenics). It takes approximately 45 min to administer. The subject is allowed to talk without interruption for 10 min, then asked a variety of questions including abstract (Why do people believe in God?), concrete (How far did you go in school?), impersonal (What do you think of President Nixon? – Reagan, Bush ...) and personal (Tell me about your first sexual experience?).

The interview is taped and afterwards rated for the presence and severity of 18 phenomena (poverty of speech, poverty of content of speech, pressure of speech, distractible speech, tangentiality, derailment, incoherence, illogicality, clanging, neologisms, word approximations, circumstantiality, loss of goal, perseveration, echolalia, blocking, stilted speech, self-reference).

All these phenomena are defined in the article and examples given.

Reliability and validity
The interview was given by its originator to manics, depressives and acute schizophrenics. inter-rater reliability was above 0.6 (weighted Kappa) for 12 of the 18 phenomena. Of these phenomena only pressure of speech, poverty of content

of speech, distractible speech and circumstantiality significantly distinguished schizophrenics from manics. Some of the phenomena were very rare in any group.

Utility
It is, in my view, a useful comprehensive assessment of the clinical phenomena, particularly in schizophrenia. Its strengths are the appreciation that thought disorder is a heterogeneous entity and the realization that manics are difficult to distinguish from schizophrenics. In addition, it provides clear definitions of the individual phenomena.

Thought Disorder Index (TDI)
(Johnston and Holzman, 1979)

The index measures degree and quality of thought disorder in psychotic subjects. It takes an hour to administer, excluding transcription time. Subjects are given the Rorschach test and their replies to each picture taped and then transcribed. The rater then looks for the presence or absence of 23 categories of thought disorder. These are divided into four groups of different degrees of severity. There are 8 at the 0.25 level, e.g. looseness; 4 at the 0.75 level, e.g. fluidity, absurd responses; and 3 at the 1.0 level, e.g. contaminations, neologisms, incoherence. A global rating between 0 and 1.0 is then made, taking into account the individual ratings.

Reliability and validity
inter-rater reliability is claimed to be good – $r = 0.9$. Holzman *et al.* (1986) claimed that manics and schizophrenics could be distinguished on the pattern of the various categorical abnormalities. Schizophrenics, they claimed, were characterized by "fluid thinking, interpenetration of one idea by another, unstable verbal referents and overly concise and contracted communications". Manics tended to have a "playful, mirthful and breezy quality" to their speech along with "loosely tied together ideas that are excessively and immoderately combined and elaborated and intrusions of incongruous ideas into social discourse".

Utility
If the claims made for this are correct it should be a useful instrument. As yet, there is no independent evaluation.

Assessment of Bizarre-idiosyncratic Thinking
(Harrow and Quinlan, 1985)

This is a global rating of thought disorder for use primarily with schizophrenics. It takes approximately 30 min to administer. Twelve questions from the comprehension subtest of the Wechsler Adult Intelligence Scale and 12 proverbs are asked. Each answer is scored 0-3 for the presence of 11 abnormalities – peculiar word form or use, lack of shared communication, coherent but odd ideas, deviant with respect to social convention, illogic, confused ideas, over-elaborated, inter-mingled, attention to limited part of stimulus, lack of relationship to stimulus material and associated inappropriate behaviour. An overall rating is then made by deriving a mean score across the 24 questions and across the 11 abnormalities.

Reliability and validity
inter-rater reliability for overall score ranged between $r = 0.67$ and $r = 0.93$ on four separate assessments. Comparison beween manics and acute schizophrenics showed no significant differences.

Utility
This procedure is only useful, in my view, for its ability to produce a single global rating. Ratings on the 11 individual abnormalities are not particularly useful, because the nature of each is not known. The procedure, therefore, might be helpful in assessing the progress of thought disorder during treatment or if correlations between thought disorder and some other phenomenon are being studied.

Formal thought Disorder Items from Schedule for Affective Disorders and Schizophrenia (SADS)
(Spitzer and Endicott, 1978) (see also Chapter 6)

This is a rapid assessment of five main types of formal thought disorder, namely incoherence, loosening of associations, illogical thinking, poverty of content of speech and neologisms in spontaneous speech. It takes only 10 min to administer.

Reliability and validity
Reliability on large samples of psychiatric patients is acceptable.

Utility
These items are useful for a quick evaluation of the varieties of thought disorder most typical of schizophrenia and as such are relatively valid indicators of schizophrenia. DSM III employs the first four of these in its criteria for schizophrenia.

Assessments and Tests of Specific Aspects of Thought Disorder

Impaired Conceptual Thinking

Similarities subtest of the Wechsler Adult Intelligence Scale
(Wechsler, 1955)
See Chapter 7 for description of the Wechsler Scale.
The Similarities subtest evaluates ability to form concepts and see relationships between things. It takes approximately 5 min to administer. The test comprises 13 pairs of words, each pair coming from the same class of items (e.g. orange, banana;

egg, seed). The subject has to say in what way the two are alike, and each response is scored 0-2 according to the criteria detailed in the test manual.

Utility
This subtest is essentially a test of verbal intelligence, but, because of the nature of the task, it may also provide a good qualitative measure of the patency or otherwise of the subject's conceptual thinking.

Whitaker Index of Schizophrenic Thinking (WIST)
(Whitaker, 1973)

This instrument assesses conceptual thinking in the context of word meanings. It takes approximately 30 min to administer.

There are 25 items, each with a stem and five multiple choice answers, all requiring a subject to select the answer which is closest in meaning to the stem. For examples Kill (stem) – (which of following is closest in meaning?) stab (too loose), cause me to die (correct), bloody me (self-reference), mill (clang), bapple (nonsense).

Reliability and validity
Reliability is excellent as it is a multiple-choice format.

Utility
Although this is a comprehensive assessment of a subject's correct knowledge of word meanings, it is not strictly a pure test of concept attainment. There is no real evidence that it is a valid test of schizophrenic thinking, despite its name.

Non-Metaphorical Thinking

The term concrete thinking is often used for the thought disorder referred to here. I prefer the term non-metaphorical thinking, partly because the terms concrete and abstract are so ambiguous, partly because numerous attempts to identify and measure "concrete thinking" have been inconclusive, and partly for theoretical reasons concerning the nature of schizophrenia – see Cutting (1990.)

Proverb Interpretation
(Gorham, 1956)

This test takes approximately 15 min to administer and involves the patient giving interpretations of 12 proverbs. Scoring varies between investigators, but it is probably best to rate each interpretation 0-3 on general adequacy.

Reliability and validity
Reliability is generally poor, in my experience. One can improve this by scrambling

the interpretations across the diagnostic groups being studied and presenting them to five normal raters who will thus be blind to the origins of the interpretations.

Utility
Most studies have found that schizophrenics give more bizarre interpretations than any other psychiatric group, though not necessarily more concrete, however this is measured. There are such individual variations, particularly in respect of intelligence, however, that the test is not a valid measure of schizophrenic thinking.

Illogical Thinking

Impaired Syllogistic Reasoning
(von Domarus, 1944)

The purpose of this test is to evaluate illogical thinking in schizophrenics. It takes approximately 10 min to administer. The precise questions used to assess syllogistic reasoning have varied between investigators. Von Domarus used strict Aristotelian syllogisms – (e.g. Stags are swift; Red Indians are swift; therefore stags are Red Indians – True? or False?) but he did not provide a list of the precise questions he used. I (Cutting and Murphy, 1988) devised 12 modern and appropriate items.

Reliability, validity and utility
There is no problem about reliability if one uses a true or false format. The validity of the procedure as a measure of schizophrenic thinking is, however, seriously in doubt. Von Domarus and others (e.g. Blanco, 1976) placed great weight on illogical thinking, measured in this way, as an index of schizophrenic thinking. Yet others (e.g. Ho, 1974; Watson and Wold, 1981) were less impressed with its usefulness in this respect.

Impaired Categorical Thinking

Overinclusive Thinking
(Epstein, 1953; Payne and Friedlander, 1962)

Several investigators have devised sorting or odd-man-out tests which they claim are reliable and valid measures of a tendency, first noted by Cameron (1939), for schizophrenics to be overinclusive in their thinking. The purpose of administering such tests is usually to confirm one's clinical impression that a schizophrenic has thought disorder. The two simplest varieties of tests for this are those devised by Epstein, and Payne and Friedlander.

Epstein's procedure
Subjects are presented with 50 stem words, each with five adjacent words which bear a greater or lesser relationship to the stem word. For example – man (stem) is

placed alongside arms, shoes, hat, toes, head, and the subject has to tick any of these five which are essential to the concept man. Overinclusive thinking is then a tendency to tick significantly more non-essential items than appropriate controls. In my study (Cutting and Murphy, 1988) I took a cut-off of two standard deviations above the mean score of mixed neurotic outpatients.

Payne and Friedlander's Procedure
They recommended presenting subjects with 12 small household objects and asking them to sort these in 10 different ways. Overinclusive thinking in this way was deemed to be present if a subject sorted according to some inessential quality of the objects concerned, e.g. scratches.

Reliability, validity and utility
The reliability of either method is questionable, as it is not clear from the literature whether the same patient will reproduce the same performance at some other time during their psychotic state. The validity of either procedure, particularly concerning the schzophrenic-manic diagnostic distinction, is also in considerable doubt. Manics are as overinclusive as schizophrenics according to Andreasen and Powers (1974), and the degree of overinclusion correlates better with the severity of a psychosis than it does with any diagnostic grouping (Davis and Blaney, 1976).

Goldstein's Sorting Tests
(Goldstein and Scheerer, 1941)

Goldstein and Scheerer devised sorting tests involving objects, woollen skeins, sticks and shapes. The purpose of these tests was to measure any impairment in the "abstract attitude", which Goldstein believed was affected in organic brain damage as well as schizophrenia. He did not provide reliability or validity measures for any of these. Rapaport (1945) tried to remedy this when he standardized the object sorting test. Thirty-three objects are to be placed in seven successive groups, the first example being chosen by the subject, the other six by the investigator. The subject is then asked to give reasons for the sorting. Abnormal responses are deemed to be present if, in the investigator's view, the group members are inappropriate.

Reliability, validity and utility
Rapaport claimed that a third of all schizophrenics will produce at least one inappropriate sort, but the general validity of this as specific to schizophrenia is still doubtful, as he had, for example, no manics.

Impaired Ability to Make Personal/Social/Emotional Judgements

Repertory Grid for Loosening of Personal Constructs
(Bannister and Fransella, 1966)

Bannister stumbled on what some, and I in particular, believe to be a core feature of schizophrenia. He noted that schizophrenics, particularly those with clinically rated thought disorder, had difficulty in rating other people consistently along some simple dimension of personality, e.g. kind, mean, etc. He devised what he called a "grid test of schizophrenic thought disorder" to measure this.

The test requires a subject to rank order eight photos of people according to how kind the subject thinks they are, then how stupid, selfish, honest, mean and sincere they seem. The subjects are then asked to repeat the whole procedure with the same eight photos for the same six traits. Two measures are derived: (1) intensity – how well ratings on one trait (e.g. kind) correlate positively with ratings on a similar trait (e.g. sincere) and negatively with those on an opposite trait (e.g. mean); (2) consistency – how well the repeat ratings correlate with the first ratings for each trait. Bannister claimed that a low intensity measure reflected loosening of a person's set of personal constructs, whereas a low consistency measure merely reflected disorganized thinking. It was the low intensity measure which he claimed was specific to schizophrenic thought disorder.

Utility
Unfortunately, the test has proved disappointing. It does not take long to administer but it takes a long time to score, as the investigator has to calculate and collate all the possible correlations. More serious, though, is the fact that schizophrenics show a low consistency score rather than a low intensity score, which simply means that their thinking is disorganized with no specific pattern to it. Furthermore, this result is not confined to schizophrenia.

Assessment of Specific Aspects of Language Disorder

The term formal thought disorder is misleading on at least two counts. First, the phenomenon which it refers to is heterogeneous in nature and the term formal thought disorders would be a better one. Second, some of the abnormalities which it covers are not strictly aspects of thinking at all. They are disorders within the realms of language and speech. In the case of schizophrenia, this "fact" is becoming more widely accepted (Wykes, 1980; Morice, 1986). However, the implications of this have not, as yet, been fully appreciated and certainly no standard tests for language disorder in any of the psychoses can be strongly recommended. The various batteries of tests used in the assessment of aphasia are unhelpful, in my view, because the pattern of language disorder in a functional psychosis is quite unlike that seen in Broca's or Wernicke's aphasia (Lecours and Vanier-Clement, 1976; Di Simoni *et al.*, 1977; Hoffman and Sledge, 1984).

There are undoubtedly abnormalities in the prosodic (Murphy and Cutting, 1990), syntactic (Morice and Ingram, 1982; Fraser *et al.*, 1986), semantic (Richman, 1968; Bar, 1976) and pragmatic (Rochester and Martin, 1979) components of schizophrenic language. Any would-be investigator of these topics will have to consult these references and devise an assessment procedure based on these studies (see Cutting, 1990, for further discussion of the issue).

Conclusions

The whole subject of thought disorder in functional psychosis is confusing. An experienced clinician can usually recognize schizophrenic thought disorder at once when he or she encounters it. But all the objective assessment procedures and tests discussed in this chapter at best only confirm this subjective impression and at worst may fail to detect what is clinically obvious. Moreover, none of them throws much light on the nature or cause of thought disorder.

Taking the assessment procedures and tests as a whole, I would recommend Andreasen's Thought, Language and Communication Scale for a comprehensive evaluation of the clinical varieties and Spitzer and Endicott's five SADS items for a quick record of the presence or absence of gross thought disorder. Of the extant purported measures of specific aspects of thought disorder I cannot heartily recommend any. Conceptual attainment is one of the few aspects of schizophrenic thinking which is intact (Cutting, 1985), and therefore no test of this is much use in schizophrenia, unless one wishes to demonstrate preservation of some functions. Categorization ability is definitely affected in a proportion of schizophrenics (25% in my study using the Epstein test of overinclusion – Cutting and Murphy, 1988). But the various tests of this are often measuring quite different abnormalities in this sphere of thinking and the critical deficit is not certain (Cutting *et al.*, 1987). Proverb interpretation is simple to administer but it is unreliable to score, is contaminated by intelligence and it is not clear what normal aspect of thinking it measures. The recently developed rating scales for delusions (see Chapter 3) look promising, but these need to be refined and standardized. I believe that Bannister was on the right lines when he devised his repertory grid of personal constructs, but it proved cumbersome to score and failed to achieve an acceptable standard of validity. In short, the ideal test of schizophrenic thought disorder has yet to be designed. In my view, this can only occur when the nature of the phenomenon is understood more clearly.

References

Andreasen, N.C. (1979). Thought, language and communication disorders. *Archives of General Psychiatry,* **36**, 1315-1330.

Andreasen, N.C. and Powers, P.S. (1974). Overinclusive thinking in mania and schizophrenia. *British Journal of Psychiatry,* **125**, 452-456.

Bannister, D. and Fransella, F. (1966). A grid test of schizophrenic thought disorder. *British*

Journal of Social and Clinical Psychology, **5**, 95-102.

Bar, E.S. (1976). Semiotic studies in schizophrenia and senile psychosis. *Semiotica*, **16**, 269-283.

Blanco, I.M. (1976). Basic logicomathematical structures in schizophrenia. *In* "Schizophrenia Today". (Eds D. Kemali, G. Bartholini, and D. Richter), pp. 211-233. Pergamon, Oxford.

Cameron, N. (1939). Schizophrenic thinking in a problem-solving situation. *Journal of Mental Science*, **85**, 1012-1035.

Cutting, J. (1985). "The Psychology of Schizophrenia". Churchill Livingstone, Edinburgh.

Cutting, J. (1990). "The Right Cerebral Hemisphere and Psychiatric Disorders". Oxford University Press, Oxford.

Cutting, J. and Murphy, D. (1988). Schizophrenia thought disorder. *British Journal of Psychiatry,* **152**, 310-319.

Cutting, J., David, A. and Murphy, D. (1987). The nature of overinclusive thinking in schizophrenia. *Psychopathology*, **20**, 213-219.

Davis, K.M. and Blaney, P.H. (1976). Overinclusion and self-editing in schizophrenia. *Journal of Abnormal Psychology,* **85**, 51-60.

Di Simoni, G.G., Darley, F.L. and Aronson, A.E. (1977). Patterns of dysfunction in schizophrenia patients on an apnasia test battery. *Journal of Speech and Hearing Disorders,* **42**, 498-513.

Epstein, S. (1953). Overinclusive thinking in a schizophrenic and a control group. *Journal of Consulting Psychology,* **17**, 384-388.

Fraser, W.I., King, K.M. Thomas, P. and Kendell, R.E. (1986). The diagnosis of schizophrenia by language analysis. *British Journal of Psychiatry,* **148**, 275-278.

Goldstein, K. and Scheerer, M. (1941). Abstract and concrete behaviour. *Psychological Monographs,* **53**, 1-151.

Gorham, D.R. (1956). A proverbs test for clinical and experimental use. *Psychological Reports*, **2**, 1-12.

Harrow, M. and Quinlan, D.M. (1985). "Disordered Thinking and Schizophrenic Psychopathology". Gardner, New York.

Ho, D.Y.F. (1974). Modern logic and schizophrenic thinking. *Genetic Psychology Monographs,* **89**, 145-165.

Hoffman, R.E. and Sledge, W. (1984). A microgenetic model of paragrammatisms produced by a schizophrenic speaker. *Brain and Language,* **21**, 147-173.

Holzman, P.S., Shenton, M.E. and Solovay, M.R. (1986). Quality of thought disorder in differential diagnosis. *Schizophrenia Bulletin,* **12**, 360-371.

Johnston, M.H. and Holzman, P.S. (1979). "Assessing Schizophrenic Thinking". Jossey-Bass, San Francisco.

Lecours, A.R. and Vanier-Clement, M. (1976). Schizophasia and jargonaphasia. *Brain and Language,* **3**, 516-565.

Morice, R. (1986). The structure, organization and use of language in schizophrenia. *In* "Handbook of Studies on Schizophrenia". Part 1. (Eds G.D. Burrows, T.R. Norman and G. Rubinstein). pp.131-144. Elsevier, Amsterdam.

Morice, R.D. and Ingram, J.C.L. (1982). Language analysis in schizophrenia: diagnostic implications. *Australian and New Zealand Journal of Psychiatry,* **16**, 11-21.

Murphy, D. and Cutting, J. (1990). Prosodic comprehension and expression in schizophrenia. *Journal of Neurology, Neurosurgery and Psychiatry*.

Payne, R.W. and Friedlander, D. (1962). A short battery of simple tests for measuring overinclusive thinking. *Journal of Mental Science,* **108**, 362-367.

Rapaport, D. (1945). "Diagnostic Psychological Testing". Vol. 1. Year Book Publishers, Chicago.

Richman, J. (1968). Symbolic distortion in the vocabulary definitions of schizophrenics. *In* "Language Behavior in Schizophrenia". (Ed. H.J. Vetter), pp. 49-57. Charles C. Thomas, Springfield.

Rochester, S.R. and Martin, J.R. (1979). "Crazy Talk". Plenum, New York.

Spitzer, R.L. and Endicott, J. (1978). "Schedule for Affective Disorders and Schizophrenia". New York State Psychiatric Institute, New York.

von Domarus, E. (1944). The specific laws of logic in schizophrenia. *In* "Language and Thought in Schizophrenia". (Ed. J.S. Kasanin), pp. 104-114. University of California Press, Berkeley.

Watson, C.G. and Wold, J. (1981). Logical reasoning deficits in schizophrenia and brain damage. *Journal of Clinical Psychology*, **37**, 466-471.

Wechsler, D. (1955). "Wechsler Adult Intelligence Scale Manual". Psychological Corporation, New York.

Whitaker, L.C. (1973). "The Whitaker Index of Schizophrenic Thinking". Western Psychological Services, Los Angeles.

Wykes, T. (1980). Language and schizophrenia. *Psychological Medicine,* **10**, 403-406.

5. The Assessment of Negative Symptoms

Thomas R. E. Barnes

The Clinical Assessment of Negative Symptoms

Sommers (1985) wrote that negative symptoms "by their very nature, represent arguably the most difficult class of clinical phenomena to measure with acceptable validity and reliability". A basic problem is that negative symptoms represent the relative absence of elements within the normal repertoire of human behaviour or function, such as emotional responsiveness, spontaneous speech and volition (Strauss *et al.*, 1974). Thus, given the difficulties of defining the limits of normality, operational definitions are difficult to generate (Sommers, 1985; Johnstone, 1989). Also, when attempting to quantify negative symptoms, rating of severity must, by definition, be on a continuum from normal. Determining the point along such a continuum that reflects the presence of pathology is likely to be arbitrary (Barnes, 1989). Thus, when attempting to assess the presence and severity of negative symptoms, raters will tend to refer back to their own experience and clinical intuition. Their ratings will be influenced by the extent of their exposure to the full range of severity of negative symptoms in patients and the normal, cultural variation in characteristics such as emotional responsiveness and expressive gesture amongst the general population.

There is a general agreement in the literature that flattened affect and poverty of speech are the core negative symptoms, a consensus that Pogue-Geile and Harrow (1988) considered to be based "mainly on convention and tradition rather than any explicit rationale". Nevertheless, these core features have consistently emerged together as part of a negative syndrome factor in factor analytic studies of symptoms of psychotic illness (Barnes and Liddle, 1990).

Assessment of these core symptoms usually relies upon observation of the patient while being interviewed by the rater. However, many patients with chronic psychotic illness will be unforthcoming and withdrawn in such circumstances, particularly if the interviewer is unfamiliar to them, as they feel anxious and uncertain or suspicious. In such cases, the rater may obtain a false impression of the patient, leading to overestimation of these negative symptoms. Further, patients may be relatively intolerant of a long interview, no matter how skilled and sympathetic the interviewer. If only a brief interview is possible initially, this is unlikely to allow the rater the opportunity to elicit the patient's full social range of emotional and verbal responses, and assessment on more than one occasion may be necessary to obtain a true picture. Apparent blunting of affect needs to be tested by the rater smiling or making a humorous remark that would be expected to elicit a smile in a normal individual. Such a strategy is explicit in the instructions for the rating of the Affective non-responsivity item of the Scale for the Assessment of Negative Symptoms (SANS) (Andreasen, 1989a,b). Some of the scales for negative symptoms include items that rate levels of social interaction, drive and interest. When using such scales, a problem may arise when attempting to collect comparable data on patient groups in different environments. For example, if studying both inpatients and outpatients, some account must be taken of the marked differences between these two groups in terms of the expectations for social behaviour and the range of opportunities for daily activities.

Distinguishing Primary Negative Symptoms

The evidence suggests that negative symptoms, as a reflection of basic deficit, constitute a valid, discrete syndrome, at least in schizophrenia (Barnes and Liddle, 1990). Nevertheless, for clinicians and researchers, a major problem in the assessment of primary negative symptoms is to distinguish them from secondary negative symptoms as a manifestation of positive symptoms, depression or the adverse effects of medication. Often, the differentiation between primary and secondary negative symptoms cannot be made at a single, clinical assessment. However, the distinction may be possible with longitudinal study, where the pattern of relationships between negative symptoms and extrapyramidal symptoms, positive psychotic symptoms and depressive features is monitored over time.

Negative Symptoms as a Manifestation of Psychosis

Carpenter *et al.* (1985) described secondary negative symptoms occurring in response to positive psychotic symptoms. They suggested that an increase in negative symptoms accompanying an exacerbation of psychosis is a common clinical observation. The explanation for such an association might be, for example, that psychotic disorganization, paranoid fears or an autistic preoccupation with hallucinatory experiences impair a patient's capacity to interact socially. Another possible mechanism is that emotional and social withdrawal may serve a defensive function, reducing the level of external stimulation for psychotic patients whose cognitive and perceptual processes are dysfunctional and overwhelmed (Carpenter *et al.*, 1985; McGlashan *et al.*, 1976). Discrimination between primary and secondary negative symptoms may be particularly relevant in patients during acute psychotic episodes.

Overlap Between Negative Symptoms and Depressive Features

The association between depressive symptoms and certain negative symptoms, such as anhedonia, anergia, feelings of emptiness and emotional withdrawal remains unclear (Stern *et al.*, 1972; McGlashan and Carpenter, 1976). For example, while some scales limit the assessment of negative symptoms to items for flattened affect and poverty of speech, others broaden the concept to include symptoms such as social withdrawal and poverty of speech, features that are common to depressive illness. For example, in two studies of chronic schizophrenic patients (Barnes *et al.*, 1989; McKenna *et al.*, 1989) depression was rated using the Montgomery-Asberg Depression Rating Scale (MADRS) (Montgomery and Asberg, 1979) and negative symptoms were scored on the SANS. While the results of both studies suggest that negative symptoms, particularly affective flattening, are separable from depression, some overlap between the scales was detected. This may be due to the inclusion in the SANS of items for anhedonia and poverty of speech, both of which are part of the clinical picture of depression.

Using the rating instruments currently available for the assessment of depression and negative symptoms, a number of studies have examined samples of schizophrenic patients to test whether negative symptoms represent a syndrome distinct from other psychotic symptoms, particularly depressive features. For example, Newcomer *et al.* (1990) administered the BPRS and the Hamilton Rating Scale for Depression (HRSD) (Hamilton, 1960) in a sample of 69 unmedicated schizophrenic inpatients. While the depression subscale of the BPRS showed a high correlation with the HRSD, the negative symptom subscale of the BPRS was unrelated to the BPRS and HRSD summary measures of depression. These authors concluded that these standard rating scales allowed negative and depressive symptoms to be assessed independently.

The results from a host of similar studies (Pogue-Geile and Harrow 1984; Iager *et al.*, 1985; Craig *et al.*, 1985; Kay *et al.*, 1986; Prosser *et al.*, 1987; House *et al.*, 1987; Whiteford *et al.*, 1987; Barnes *et al.*, 1989; McKenna *et al.*, 1989) predominantly suggest that blunted or flattened affect, particularly, is clinically distinguishable from depression. For example, in a group of schizophrenic out-patients, Prosser *et al.* (1987) found no association between scores on the HRSD and the BPRS negative symptom subscale. While a significant correlation was found between the BPRS subscale and items from the HRSD reflecting "vegetative" features of depression (decreased work and activities, motor retardation and decreased libido), suggesting that such features may be common to both depression and the negative syndrome, there was no such positive correlation between negative symptoms and "cognitive" features of depression (depressed mood, suicidal idea-tion and guilt). The investigators concluded that, within their patient sample, flattened affect was distinguishable from depressed affect.

To examine further the overlap between depressive symptoms and negative symptoms, Siris *et al.* (1988) studied a sample of 46 patients with syndromes of post-psychotic depression following episodes of schizophrenia or schizoaffective disorder. All the patients were receiving depot antipsychotic medication and anticholinergic drugs. Twenty-three of these depressed schizophrenic or schizoaffective patients also fulfilled the definition for a negative syndrome. But, in terms of severity of depressive symptoms, the subgroup meeting the criteria for a negative syndrome did not differ significantly from the remaining 23 patients who did not. The authors considered this evidence that the negative syndrome differs from post-psychotic depression qualitatively rather than just quantitatively.

Negative Symptoms Secondary to Antipsychotic Drug Effects

Uncontrolled studies have consistently failed to find any significant positive relationship between negative symptoms and dosage of antipsychotic medication (Pogue-Geile and Zubin, 1988). For example, in a controlled study, Brier and colleagues (1987) found that withdrawal of antipsychotic medication exacerbated negative symptoms while reinstitution of drug treatment improved them. Further, a study comparing relatively young schizophrenic patients on and off antipsychotic medication (Pogue-Geile and Harrow, 1985) revealed no significant differences in negative symptom scores. These findings suggest that ratings of negative symptoms are not primarily a reflection of side-effects of antipsychotic drug treatment.

Nevertheless, there may be a genuine difficulty in distinguishing clinically between certain features of drug-induced parkinsonism and negative symptoms (Prosser *et al.*, 1987). The rating of schizophrenic affect requires a subtle consideration of facial mobility and expressiveness (Corradi, 1978; Reid *et al.*, 1982). Thus, the assessment of negative symptoms is likely to be seriously confounded by the presence of drug-induced parkinsonism, particularly the bradykinesia component with features such a lack of facial expression, loss of spontaneity and paucity of gesture.

The Assessment Procedures

Nonspecific Rating Scales

Brief Psychiatric Rating Scale (BPRS)
(Overall and Gorham 1962)(see Chapter 2 for fuller description, also Chapters 3 and 6)

The BPRS negative symptom subscale (NSS) is composed of the items rating emotional withdrawal, motor retardation and blunted affect. This subscale was originally referred to as a "withdrawal-retardation" factor, emerging as one of four higher-order factors when the full scale was subjected to factor analysis (Overall, 1974). However, other investigators have selected emotional withdrawal, uncooperativeness and blunted affect as the negative items of the BPRS (Eccleston *et al.*, 1985).

Reliability and validity
Thiemann *et al.* (1987) tested the inter-rater reliability of the NSS alone in a sample

of 30 patients with a diagnosis of schizophrenia. Using the Spearman rank correlation coefficient, the reliability was 0.81. In a separate sample of 35 male patients with a diagnosis of either schizophrenia or schizoaffective disorder, the inter-rater reliabilities of the SANS and the NSS were tested, with both scales being completed for each interview. Using the scales together, the inter-rater reliability for the NSS was 0.73 compared with 0.69 for the SANS composite score.

Thiemann *et al.* (1987) also investigated the factor structure of the full BPRS using a principal components analysis. This revealed a factor structure similar to that originally found by Overall (1974) with the three items of the withdrawal-retardation subscale showing a strong intercorrelation.

Utility
Kay (1991) points out that the three negative items comprising the NSS show a differential response to antipsychotic medication (Angrist *et al.*, 1980) which suggests that they are conceptually distinct, and challenges the validity of combining them in a subscale. Andreasen (1990) makes the general criticism that the BPRS (see Chapter 2, page 12) was developed through factor analysis and rates at the relatively abstract level of factors rather than symptoms. Clinically-trained raters may find the scale difficult to apply, being more familiar with the assessment of mental state phenomena in terms of specific symptoms.

Manchester Scale (MS)
(Krawiecka et al., 1977) (see also Chapters 2, 3 and 6)

This scale, also referred to as the Krawiecka, or Krawiecka and Goldberg scale, was designed for the brief rating of chronic psychotic patients by doctors who know them well (see Chapter 2, page 16). It is reviewed in some detail here as it has been commonly used in studies of negative symptoms (Crow, 1985). Johnstone and her colleagues (1978) subdivided the scale into positive, negative and non-specific, sub-scales of schizophrenia. These investigators also separated flattened affect and incongruous affect which are combined in one item in the original scale. The negative symptom subscale consists of only two items, flattening (but not incongruity) of affect and poverty of speech. Both items are rated on a five-point scale of severity (0-4). A rating of 1 suggests some evidence for the presence of the symptom, but this is not considered pathological. A rating of 2 refers to a degree of severity just sufficient to be pathological while ratings of 3 or 4 refer to marked and severe psychopathology, respectively.

Reliability and validity
A new rater can partially train himself by using available training videotapes, from the Department of Psychiatry, University of Manchester, and establish his reliability by using additional videotapes especially prepared for this purpose (Hyde, 1989). Manchanda and Hirsch (1979, unpublished) modified the manual by introducing a series of questions derived from the PSE in order to facilitate

interviewing and provide adequate coverage of symptoms seen in acute patients.

Krawiecka, Goldberg and Vaughan (1977) carried out reliability testing of the scale and produced satisfactory levels of inter-rater reliability with five psychiatrists rating from videotapes and patient interviews. Ratings based on a verbal report had a correlation coefficient ranging from 0.75 - 0.87, except for anxiety for which the figure was around 0.65. The corresponding range for items based on observation was 0.62 - 0.73, except for flattened or incongruous affect where the figures were between 0.50 and 0.58. Further, there were no differences between the raters in their mean severity scores except for the flattened/incongruous affect item. In another study (Manchanda et al., 1986) the BPRS and MS were used by two raters from different cultures and different educational backgrounds (Indian psychiatrist and German psychologist / medical student) without any previous experience in the use of the two scales. The correlation coefficients for the majority of the items on the MS were higher than those for the BPRS. A higher inter-rater reliability for items on the MS was seen whether patients were rated at the same or different points in time by the two raters. Vaughan and Krawiecka (1979) examined the sensitivity of the scale in patients with chronic schizophrenia, the group for which the scale was devised. The scale was tested under conditions comparable to a controlled treatment trial, with a sample of 34 patients being rated on three occasions. The investigators found that the scale was sensitive to change in the severity of psychotic symptoms. Further, analysis of the intercorrelations of the eight scale items over the three occasions yielded two enduring clusters of symptoms. One of these comprised the three items rating negative symptoms: flattened or incongruous affect; mutism; and psychomotor retardation.

Jackson et al. (1990) carried out an investigation of the psychometric properties of the MS in a sample of 53 schizophrenic patients. Factor analysis of the eight scale items revealed that only the negative symptoms were related to one other. The negative symptoms were strongly correlated with the SANS, suggesting good concurrent validity for the MS negative subscale.

Utility

The MS and the negative subscale has been used not only for the assessment of patients with chronic psychotic illness (Owens and Johnstone, 1980; Johnstone et al., 1986) but also as a measure of change in acute treatment trials (Johnstone et al., 1978a). The investigators have found it brief, simple to use and sensitive to change. Hyde (1989) suggest that the scale is appropriate for use in drug trials, rehabilitation studies and the assessment of large populations of chronic patients, including multicentre population comparisons.

The disadvantages of the scale are, first, a lack of items covering features of mania, such as elevated mood and overactivity. Second, there is possibly some lack of sensitivity for rating the severity of certain symptoms. On the five-point scale, the presence of indubitably pathological features may warrant a rating of 3, allowing only one possible higher rating for greater severity.

Specific Rating Scales for Negative Symptoms

Scale for the Assessment of Negative Symptoms (SANS)
(Andreasen 1981, 1989a,b) (see also Chapter 8)

The Scale for Assessment of Positive Symptoms (SAPS) and the Scale for Assessment of Negative Symptoms (SANS) were designed as part of a psychiatric assessment battery known as the Comprehensive Assessment of Symptoms and History (CASH), covering medical history, neurological examination and social data. The positive and negative symptom scales were designed to provide a comprehensive assessment of the symptoms of schizophrenia and to measure their change over time (Andreasen 1985, 1989a).

The items on the SANS are primarily observational items, one basic assumption in the development of the scale being that reliability is best achieved through the use of such an approach, rather than by probing the patient's internal psychological state (Andreasen 1989a). The scale comprises five subgroups of negative features: Alogia, including poverty of speech, poverty of content of speech, blocking and increased speech latency; Affective flattening, including unchanging facial expression, decreased spontaneous movements, paucity of expressive gestures, affective non-responsivity and inappropriate affect; Avolition-Apathy, including impersistence at work and school and physical anergia; Anhedonia-Asociality, including ratings of sexual interest and activity and ability to feel intimacy and closeness; and Attention, which includes social inattentiveness. Originally, the scale included items requiring patient reports of their awareness and experience of negative symptoms, such as subjective complaints of emotional emptiness or loss of feeling, and subjective complaints of inattentiveness. However, these items have been found to correlate poorly with the other symptoms in each subgroup (Andreasen, 1982; Thiemann *et al.*, 1987) and have been dropped from recent versions of the scale (Andreasen, 1989b).

Reliability and validity
The reliability of the SANS has been repeatedly tested in a variety of cultural settings. Andreasen (1989a) presented data from studies conducted in the USA Japan (Ohta *et al.*, 1984), Italy (Moscarelli *et al.*, 1987) and Spain (Humbert *et al.*, 1986), revealing a consistently high level of reliability for the global ratings. Andreasen stresses the value of adequate training in achieving good reliability, and has developed training materials for the SANS, including videotapes and case vignettes, that have been widely used in America.

Andreasen (1989a) has presented data from two separate replication studies, involving over 150 schizophrenic patients, showing that the items within each of these five categories constitute valid symptom groupings, that is, show high internal consistency. Analysis using Cronbach's alpha revealed that the individual items used to make the global ratings are highly intercorrelated. Further, the five global ratings are also highly correlated with one another, the coefficient alpha ranging from 0.63 to 0.83. Thiemann *et al.* (1987) confirmed this good internal consistency for the SANS, with Cronbach's alpha values from 0.67 to 0.90 for the five subscales. They also carried out a principal components analysis on the global ratings for the five subscales and found a single factor which accounted for 58% of the total variance on these items. They concluded that there was a unitary dimension of negative symptoms underlying the five symptom complexes.

Walker *et al.* (1988) confirmed the significant intercorrelation of negative symptoms within the SANS in schizophrenic patients, with the exception of affective flattening and attentional impairment. The latter symptom was positively correlated with severity of thought disorder and total positive symptom score, a finding consistent with other reports (Bilder *et al.*, 1985; Cornblatt *et al.*, 1985; Gur *et al.*, 1991). The authors also challenged the validity of the attentional impairment item on the basis that they had found no association between attentional deficits on a digit span task and observer ratings of attentional impairment during an interview (Walker and Harvey, 1986).

The SANS has been found to correlate well with the BPRS negative symptom items (Thiemann *et al.*, 1987; Czobor *et al.*, 1991) and the negative scale of the PANSS (Kay, 1991) suggesting good concurrent validity for the scale.

Utility

The symptoms and signs covered by the SANS items are not specific to schizophrenia, and Andreasen (1989*a*) noted that the scale could be used to observe the frequency of these features in a variety of diagnostic categories. For example, elements of anhedonia, alogia and impaired social functioning referred to in the scale are also recognized manifestations of a depressive illness. This raises the question of whether the presence of depressive features in schizophrenic patients will confound the rating of negative symptoms on the SANS. Within samples of schizophrenic patients, studies using established rating scales such as the SANS, BPRS, and the Hamilton Rating Scale for Depression have generally demonstrated that depressive features and negative symptoms are largely separable and discrete domains of pathology (see Barnes and Liddle, 1990), although there is some overlap in pathology.

Dworkin (1990) used the SANS in a study of 220 schizophrenic twins and interpreted the results as suggesting that negative symptoms and disordered social relationships were manifestations of distinct processes in the development of schizophrenia. He concluded that items assessing asociality should be excluded from rating scales for negative symptoms.

Positive and Negative Syndrome Scale (PANSS)
(Kay et al., 1986; Kay, 1991) (see also Chapter 3)

The use of the PANSS (see also Chapter 3, page 26) involves a 30-40 min formalized psychiatric interview. A detailed rating manual is available (Kay *et al.*, 1986) which contains guidelines for the interview, including suggested questions for probing particular areas of psychopathology. Subsequently, a more detailed structured interview has been developed to obtain information relevant to diagnostic criteria as well as the assessment of schizophrenic symptoms. This Structured Clinical Interview for the DSM-III-R, PANSS edition (SCID-PANSS) includes a pre-interview which gathers information on the patient's functioning from care workers or relatives, as well as a structured interview with the patient (Kay, 1991).

For each item, a definition of the symptom is provided as well as detailed criteria for each rating level, from 1 (absent) to 7 (extreme). Scores from 2 to 7 rate severity, on the criteria of the prominence of the symptom, frequency during the observation period and the degree of interference with functioning.

As reflected in the title of this scale, the originators subscribed to the notion of two phenomenologically distinct syndromes within schizophrenia (Kay and Opler, 1987). Of the 30 items included in the PANSS, seven constitute a negative subscale (NS). Two of these, blunted affect and emotional withdrawal, derive from the BPRS. The five new items are poor rapport, passive/apathetic social withdrawal, difficulty in abstract thinking, lack of spontaneity and flow of conversation and stereotyped thinking.

Reliability and validity
High inter-rater reliability and test-retest reliablity have been demonstrated for the scale (Kay *et al.*, 1987, 1988; Kay, 1991). To examine the internal consistency of the PANSS, Kay *et al.* (1987) applied Cronbach's coefficient alpha to the data from a sample of 101 chronic schizophrenic inpatients. Each of the items in the NS showed a strong correlation with the total ($p < 0.001$), and, overall, the internal reliability (alpha coefficient) was 0.83.

Inter-rater reliability was tested in a sample of young, acute schizophrenia patients (Kay *et al.*, 1988). Two psychologists and one psychiatrist rated the PANSS on the basis of the same interview. The inter-rater concordance was examined statistically using the Pearson correlation. The mean Pearson correlation for the NS was 0.85 ($p < 0.0001$), a correlation which, Kay (1991) noted, compared favourably with those reported for other similar symptom scales.

In addition, the PANSS shows a close correspondence with the Andreasen scales, SAPS and SANS, which Kay *et al.* (1988) present as a demonstration of criterion-related validity for the scale. Particularly, the negative syndrome of the PANSS was found to be highly correlated with the SANS. Further, the positive and negative syndrome subscales were found to be significantly inversely related, after adjustment for the overall level of severity of the illness, as measured by the general psychopathology subscale. The authors took this finding as an illustration of the mutually exclusive nature of the positive and negative syndrome ratings, and evidence for the construct validity of the subscales.

Utility

Most of the items on the NS are rated on the basis of a patient's responses and interpersonal behaviour during the standard interview. However, ratings of emotional withdrawal should take account of reports of functioning from "primary care workers or family" and ratings on the item for passive/apathetic social withdrawal are based entirely on such reports.

Of the core negative symptoms, blunted affect and poverty of speech, the latter is not rated directly on the NS, but rather as a component of the items for poor rapport and lack of spontaneity and flow of conversation. The items for stereotyped thinking and lack of spontaneity both refer to restricted communication during the interview, and if this is present, the rater must make a judgement regarding the relevant psychological mechanisms in order to score the correct item. While restriction of a patient's communication due to apathy, avolition, defensiveness or cognitive deficit should be rated on the lack of spontaneity item, restriction of communication due to rigid thinking, repetition or barren thought content is rated under the item for stereotyped thinking. Thus, the item for stereotyped thinking seems to incorporate the concept of poverty of content of speech, as included, for example, in the SANS.

The lack of flexibility rated on the item for stereotyped thinking refers to the conversation being limited to two or three dominating topics. If these recurrent topics referred to delusional ideas with which the patient is preoccupied, the rating would essentially reflect a secondary negative symptom.

The Psychological Impairments Rating Scale (PIRS)
(Jablensky et al., 1980; Biehl et al., 1989a,b)

Behavioural Observation Schedule (BOS)
(Atakan and Cooper, 1989)

The PIRS was originally designed to serve as a supplement to the PSE in a number of WHO collaborative studies. It rates observed behaviour, and represents an elaboration of the final sections of the PSE covering behaviour, affect and speech (Jablensky *et al.*, 1980; Biehl *et al.*, 1989a).

The total schedule contains 97 items divided into 10 sections. Four of these sections, that is, slowness/"psychic tempo", attention/withdrawal, fatiguability and initiative are grouped under the title activity/withdrawal, while the other six sections, communication by facial expression, communication by body language, affect display, conversation skills, self-presentation and cooperation are grouped as ratings of social skills. Each section has an overall impression item rated from 0 (no disturbance) to 5 (maximum disturbance).

Recently, the PIRS has been revised in response to a number of perceived problems (Atakan and Cooper, 1989). First, there was apparently a need for more detailed rating instructions and more precise definitions for many of the scale items. Second, there was possibly some overlap between some of the items, in that they might be rating the same behaviour. Third, certain common aspects of observed behaviour were thought to be missing from the schedule. Lastly, the scale was considered to require reorganization so that the general order of the items corresponded more closely to the routine, clinical examination of the mental state. The authors claim that the new version, named the Behavioural Observation Schedule (BOS), includes observed behaviours seen in a wider range of psychiatric disorder than just the functional psychoses. The BOS consists of five main sections: self-presentation; activity; display of affect; communication skills; and co-operation.

Reliability and validity
Extensive training, involving both clinical interviews and prepared videotapes may be necessary to achieve an adequate level of inter-rater reliability (Biehl *et al.*, 1989*b*). Nevertheless, on the basis of 58 interviews, Biehl *et al.* (1989*b*) reported a kappa of 0.79 and a pairwise agreement rate of 89.4%. No detailed psychometric information is available for the BOS, but Atakan and Cooper (1989) reported good reliability between two observers, rating 20 videotaped PSE interviews.

Utility
Over the last decade, the PIRS scale has been used in many studies, particularly in the context of the WHO Mental Health Programme. For example, Biehl *et al.* (1988) used the PIRS to assess impairment in a prospective, five-year study of a cohort of 70 first-onset schizophrenic patients. In this, as in most studies, the scale was employed in combination with a semi-structured interview, such as the PSE.

The High Royds Evaluation of Negativity (HEN)
(Mortimer et al., 1989)

This new scale (Mortimer *et al.*, 1989) was designed to be quick and easy to use, without the need for an informant. It places particular emphasis on the objective rating of disturbance of affect, with items for constricted affect, emotional withdrawness and shallow/coarsened affect. The description of this last symptom includes a caution to raters not to confuse it with inappropriate affect.

The scale comprises 18 symptom ratings divided into six categories: appearance; behaviour; speech; thought; affect; and general functioning. Each symptom is rated from 0 (absent) to 4 (severe). In addition, there is a global score item for each category and a summary score consisting of the sum of the six global scores.

Reliability and validity
Good inter-rater reliability has been demonstrated (Mortimer *et al.*, 1989). Con-

struct (convergent) validity was suggested by a strong correlation with blindly rated items on the Social Behaviour Schedule (Wykes and Sturt, 1986) related to negativity, but none with items representing positive symptoms. HEN scale ratings were also independent of measures of mood, arguing for a degree of construct (divergent) validity.

The Negative Symptom Rating Scale (NSRS)
(Iager et al., 1985)

The NSRS is a relatively short scale for rating negative symptoms in schizophrenia (Iager *et al.*, 1985). Each item is rated on a 7-point scale from 0 (normal) to 6 (severely impaired). While the scale covers symptoms included in other scales for negative symptoms, such as a lack of emotional response and amount of coherent speech, it also addresses less usual features such as the patient's ability to make decisions and judgements, and expressive relatedness, described as "the spontaneity, amount and sincerity of interactions between the patient and others...". Also included in the scale are tests of cognitive functioning, with items for rating memory impairment, attention and orientation. Volition and motivation are assessed with items for grooming and self care, degree of supervision and help required for tasks of daily living and the amount and speed of voluntary body movement.

Reliability and validity
Iager *et al.* (1985) demonstrated acceptable inter-rater reliability for the individual scale items, with weighted kappa ranging from 0.57 for grooming to 0.97 for memory. The reliability was improved by grouping items into subscale totals, and the intraclass correlation coefficient for total scale scores was 0.96 ($p < 0.0001$). These authors also tested the construct validity of the NSRS by investigating its correlation with the SANS, BPRS, MS and the Emotional Blunting Scale of Abrams and Taylor (1978). The highest correlation was between the NSRS and the SANS, although there were also reasonable correlations with the other scales despite their differences in item contents.

The Schedule for the Deficit Syndrome (SDS)
(Kirkpatrick et al., 1989)

The SDS is an instrument designed to categorize schizophrenic patients into those with and those without the deficit syndrome. The deficit syndrome is a schizophrenic subtype delineated by Carpenter *et al.* (1985). The diagnostic criteria include the presence of two or more negative symptoms out of the following six: restricted affect; diminished emotional range; poverty of speech; curbing of interests; diminished sense of purpose; and diminished social drive. The negative symptoms must be primary, and persistent during the patient's periods of clinical stability.

The six negative symptoms are described in more detail by Kirkpatrick *et al.* (1989). They are each rated on a five-point scale (0-4), with a rating of 2 representing a symptom that is "clearly pathological". A manual for the SDS is available on request from its authors, and this provides guidelines for the interview of patients and the collection of relevant information.

Reliability and validity
Kirkpatrick *et al.* (1989) reported inter-rater reliability data for the scale. Employing the guidelines for the SDS contained in the manual, two raters assessed 40 schizophrenic patients using the scale. The unweighted kappa value for the global deficit vs nondeficit categorization was 0.73, reflecting agreement on the classification in 36 of the cases. Weighted kappa values were also given for the six negative symptoms, and ranged from 0.6 for diminished social drive to 0.74 for restricted affect.

Kirkpatrick *et al.* (1989) also collected SDS data from a larger sample of 70 patients and analyzed these to test the cohesiveness of the deficit syndrome construct. They calculated the rank-order correlations of each negative symptom with the other five, using Spearman's rho. The correlations were relatively high, ranging from 0.47 between curbing of interests and diminished emotional range to a value of 0.84 for the correlation between restricted affect and poverty of speech.

The Negative Symptom Assessment (NSA)
(Alphs et al., 1989a,b)

Alphs and his colleagues developed the NSA to overcome what they considered to be serious deficiencies of the available scales of negative symptoms. The scale covers a broad range of negative symptoms, comprising 27 items within six categories: communication; emotion/affect; social activity; motivation; cognition and psychomotor activity. In addition, there is an item for rating global severity. Each item is rated on a six-point scale (1-6), indicating absent, questionable, mild, moderate, marked and severe symptoms respectively. The total NSA score represents the sum of the scores for the 27 individual items.

Reliability and validity
One hundred patients, with a diagnosis of either schizophrenia or schizoaffective disorder, were interviewed using a semi-structured questionnaire designed to elicit the information necessary to complete the NSA, SANS and BPRS negative symptom subscale (Alphs *et al.*, 1989a). These interviews were videotaped.

Four observers rated 66 of the videotaped interviews and completed the three scales. Inter-rater reliability was examined, and the correlation coefficients obtained with the NSA were reported to be comparable with those obtained with the SANS and BPRS subscale. To test intrarater reliability, observers rated the same interview on two occasions, at least two weeks apart. To evaluate occasion reliability, ratings of the same videotaped interview were compared. In order to evaluate the reliability between live and videotape ratings, the ratings of a live interview were compared with a later rating of the same interview on videotape.

Construct validity was determined by a principal components analysis with varimax rotation of the data from the total patient sample. Seven factors were generated, labelled by the authors as affect/emotion, external involvement, retardation, personal presentation, thinking, interpersonal interest and blocking. The authors note that while these component factors require independent evaluation, they do not support the use of the original six categories for data analysis.

To establish concurrent validity for the NSA, the relationships between the NSA, SANS and BPRS subscale were examined. High correlations between the total scale scores were found. For example, there was a correlation of 0.8 between NSA and BPRS subscale total scores while the figure for NSA and SANS scores was 0.9.

Subjective Experience of Deficits in Schizophrenia (SEDS)
(Liddle and Barnes, 1988) (see also Chapter 8)

This scale was designed principally to measure the subjective experience of negative symptoms, that is, to evaluate patients' awareness of the disorganization or impoverishment of mental activity in schizophrenia which is more usually inferred from observation of behaviour. The items were partly based upon consideration of Huber's pure defect syndrome (Huber *et al.*, 1980; Gross, 1989; Roth, 1989) as interpreted by Koehler and Sauer (1984).

The SEDS consists of 21 items, each rated on a five-point scale (0-4), arranged in five groups: abnormal thinking and concentration; disturbance of affect; impaired will and decreased energy; disturbance of perception and motor function; and intolerance of stress. The individual items are defined in a glossary which is available from the authors. The ratings are made on the basis of a semi-standardized interview, with a specific probe question for each item.

Reliability and validity
In a sample of chronic, schizophrenic inpatients it proved possible to rate the various subjective experiences with satisfactory inter-rater reliability, the values of Cohen's weighted kappa ranging from 0.94 for distorted special sensation to 0.53 for distorted visceral sensation (Liddle and Barnes, 1988). The generally high level of inter-rater agreement suggested that the majority of the 52 schizophrenic inpatients in the sample were able to give a comprehensible account of their experience of deficits.

Subjective Deficit Syndrome Scale (SDSS)
(Bitter et al., 1989; Jaeger et al., 1990)

Like the SEDS, the SDSS (Bitter *et al.*, 1989) was developed for the assessment of subjective symptoms. It is based upon the Subclinical Symptoms Scale (Petho and Bitter, 1985) which represented an earlier attempt to assess the pure defect syndrome of Huber in a quantitative and standardized manner. The SDSS has 19 items which are self-rated, in that they are scored on the basis of the patient's responses to prompts or questions and the examiner's judgement about the validity or consistency of these responses has no influence on the ratings. Each item refers to a subjective complaint such as difficulties with thinking, concentration and motivation, loss of emotions and ability to feel pleasure, nervousness and irritability. The items are rated on a five-point scale (0-4), reflecting the degree of disturbance reported.

Reliability and validity
Jaeger *et al.* (1990) reported on the reliability of the SDSS in four independent samples, consisting of 166 psychiatric patients. Coefficient alpha showed good internal consistency in each of the samples, with values ranging from 0.75 to 0.87. Inter-rater reliability was highly significant, with intra-class correlation values ranging from 0.97 to 0.99. Test-retest reliability was calculated for one of the samples; 28 schizophrenic inpatients rated on two occasions, 24 hours apart. The intra-class correlation was 0.95.

Comparative Utility of Assessment Procedures

Leach (1991) asserts that there are serious doubts about the validity and reliability of the current rating instruments for negative symptoms. She states the scales are "problematic, assessing insufficient numbers of items, poorly defining or assessing more than one concept, lacking precise rating criteria, utilizing inadequate interviews, not defining the population in which they should be used, or not demonstrating subjects' changes over time." Alphs *et al.* (1989*a*) compiled a similar list of criticisms. Nevertheless, adequate inter-rater reliability has been demonstrated for most of the scales, and good correlation between the scales suggests reasonable concurrent validity.

The BPRS negative symptom subscale and the SANS are probably the most widely used scales for assessing negative symptoms. Thiemann *et al.* (1987) compared the two scales in terms of their factor structures, their inter-rater reliabilities when used alone and in combination, and the correlation between them. They concluded that, in their study, the two scales were equivalent measures of negative symptoms and their use together was therefore redundant. This issue was also explored by Czobor *et al.* (1991). These authors found the two scales to be highly intercorrelated but, analyzing the data from the two scales administered to 61 acutely psychotic schizophrenic patients, they concluded that the individual items and subscales of SANS contained independent information compared with the BPRS. However, when the SANS was represented by the single composite score, the independent information was lost and it was redundant with the anergia factor of the BPRS.

For the majority of rating scales for negative symptoms, rating of the items relies heavily on the interpretation of observed behaviour. The scales that assess the subjective complaints of patients, such as the SEDS and SDSS, would seem to be rating a different domain of psychopathology in that these ratings do not correlate with objective negative symptoms. However, some overlap with depressed mood has been reported (Liddle and Barnes, 1988; Jaeger *et al.*, 1990).

Each of the negative symptom scales described covers a broad range of features that reflects the variety of operational definitions for negative symptoms that underlie the instruments (Pogue-Geile and Zubin, 1988). While the symptoms and signs included in the various scales tend to overlap on core features such as flattened affect and poverty of speech, they can differ markedly on other features, some of which may carry a risk of overlap with other domains such as social behaviour and role performance, depression and cognitive function. For example, the SANS includes items for anhedonia and attentional impairment, while the NSRS and NSA include items rating memory deficit and disorientation.

The selection of a scale for research or clinical use will depend upon the symptoms of particular interest, but the SANS is probably the best instrument for general purposes. If it is necessary to rate only the core negative symptoms of flattened affect and poverty of speech and there is no requirement to rate neurotic or psychotic symptoms in great detail, the MS may be an appropriate scale (Manchanda *et al.*, 1989). The BPRS is also seen as a simple and reliable scale, with three items constituting a negative symptom subscale. The PANSS represents a development of the BPRS, with a negative subscale that includes two items from the BPRS and five new items.

References

Abrams, R. and Taylor, M.A. (1978). A rating scale for emotional blunting. *American Journal of Psychiatry*, **135**, 226-229.

Alphs, L.D., Summerfelt, A., Lann, H. and Muller, R.J. (1989*a*) The negative symptom assessment: a new instrument to assess negative symptoms of schizophrenia. *Psychopharmacology Bulletin,* **25**, 159-163.

Alphs, L.D., Lafferman, J.A., Ross, L., Bland, W. and Levine, J. (1989*b*). Fenfluramine treatment of negative symptoms in older schizophrenic inpatients. *Psychopharmacology Bulletin,* **25**, 149-153.

Andreasen, N.C. (1981). "The Scale for the Assessment of Negative Symptoms (SANS)". The University of Iowa, Iowa City, Iowa.

Andreasen, N.C. (1985). Positive vs. negative schizophrenia. *Schizophrenia Bulletin,* **11**, 380-389.

Andreasen, N.C. (1989*a*). Scale for the assessment of negative symptoms (SANS). *British Journal of Psychiatry,* **155** (supplement 7), 53-58.

Andreasen, N.C. (1989*b*). The scale for the assessment of negative symptoms (SANS): Conceptual and theoretical foundations. *British Journal of Psychiatry,* **155**, (supplement 7), 49-52.

Andreasen, N.C. and Olsen, S. (1982). Negative and positive schizophrenia, definition and validation. *Archives of General Psychiatry*, **39**, 789-793.

Angrist, B., Rotrosen, J. and Gershon, S. (1980). Differential effects of amphetamine and neuroleptics on negative vs. positive symptoms in schizophrenia. *Psychopharmacology*, **72**, 17-19.

Atakan, Z. and Cooper, J.E. (1989). Behavioural Observation Schedule (BOS), PIRS 2nd edition: A revised edition of the PIRS (WHO, Geneva, March 1978). *British Journal of Psychiatry*, **155**, (supplement 7), 78-80.

Barnes, T.R.E. (1989). Introduction. *British Journal of Psychiatry*, **155**, (supplement 7), 8-9.

Barnes, T.R.E. and Liddle, P.F. (1990). The evidence for the validity of negative symptoms. *In* "Modern Problems of Pharmacopsychiatry, Schizophrenia: Positive and Negative Symptoms and Syndromes". (Ed. N.C. Andreasen), pp 43-72. Karger, Basel.

Barnes, T.R.E., Curson, D.A., Liddle, P.F. and Patel, M. (1989). The nature and prevalence of depression in chronic schizophrenic inpatients. *British Journal of Psychiatry*, **154**, 486-491.

Biehl, H., Schubart, C., Jung, E. *et al.* (1988). Reported symptoms in schizophrenic patients within 5 years of onset of illness – A report from the prospective Rhine Neckar cohort study. *In* "Treatment Refractory Schizophrenia". (Ed. S.J. Dencker, W, Bender and F. Kulhanek). Braunschweig, Vieweg.

Biehl, H., Maurer, K., Jablensky, A., Cooper, J.E. and Tomov, T . (1989*a*). The WHO Psychological Impairments Rating Schedule (WHO/PIRS): I. Introducing a new instrument for rating observed behaviour and the rationale of the psychological impairments concept. *British Journal of Psychiatry,* **155** (supplement 7), 68-70.

Biehl, H., Maurer, K., Jung, E. and Krumm, B. (1989*b*). The PIRS/WHO. II. Impairments in schizophrenics in cross-sectional and longitudinal perspective. the Mannheim experience in two independent samples. *British Journal of Psychiatry,* **155**, (supplement 7), 71-77.

Bilder, R.M., Mukherjee, S., Rieder, R.O. and Pandurangi, A.K. (1985). Symptomatic and neuropsychological components of defect states. *Schizophrenia Bulletin*, **11**, 409-419.

Bitter, I., Jaeger, J., Agdeppa, J. and Volavka, J. (1989). Subjective symptoms: part of the negative syndrome of schizophrenia. *Psychopharmacology Bulletin,* **25**, 180-185.

Brier, A., Wolkowitz, O.M., Doran, A.R., Roy, A., Boronow, J., Hommer, D.W. and Pickar, D. (1987). Neuroleptic responsivity of negative and positive symptoms in schizophrenia. *American Journal of Psychiatry*, **144**, 1549-1555.

Carpenter, W.T., Heinrichs, D.W. and Alphs, L.D. (1985). Treatment of negative symptoms. *Schizophrenia Bulletin*, **11**, 441-452.

Cornblatt, B.A., Lenzenwager, M.F., Dworkin, R.H. and Erlemeyer-Kimling, L. (1985). Positive and negative schizophrenic symptoms. Attention and information processing. *Schizophrenia Bulletin*, **11**, 397-405.

Corradi, R.B. (1978). Clinical assessment of affect in schizophrenia. *Journal of Clinical Psychiatry*, **39**, 493-496.

Craig, T.J., Richardson, M.A., Pass, R. and Bregman, Z. (1985). Measurement of mood and affect in schizophrenic inpatients. *American Journal of Psychiatry*, **142**, 1272-7.

Crow, T.J. (1985). The two-syndrome concept: origins and current status. *Schizophrenia Bulletin*, **11**, 471-486.

Czobor, P., Bitter, I. and Volavka, J. (1991). Relationship between the Brief Psychiatric Rating Scale and the Scale for the Assessment of Negative Symptoms: a study of their correlation and redundancy. *Psychiatry Research,* **36**, 129-139.

Dworkin RH. (1990). Patterns of sex differences in negative symptoms and social functioning consistent with separate dimensions of schizophrenic pathology. *American Journal of Psychiatry*, **147**, 347-349.

Eccleston, D., Fairbairn, A.F., Hassanyeh, F., McClelland, H.A. and Stephens, D.A. (1985). The effect of propranolol and thioridazine on positive and negative symptoms of schizophrenia. *British Journal of Psychiatry*, **147**, 623-630.

Gur, R.E., Mozley, P.D., Resnick, S.M., Levick, S., Erwin, R., Saykin., A.J. and Gur, R.C. (1991). Relations among clinical scales in schizophrenia. *American Journal of Psychiatry*, **148**, 472-478.

Gross, G. (1989). The "basic" symptoms of schizophrenia. *British Journal of Psychiatry*, **155**, (supplement 7), 21-25.

Hamilton, M. (1960). Rating scale for depression. *Journal of Neurology, Neurosurgery and Psychiatry*, **23**, 56-62.

House, A., Bostock, J., Cooper, J. (1987). Depressive symptoms in the year following onset of a first schizophrenic episode. *British Journal of Psychiatry*, **151**, 773-779.

Huber, G., Gross, G., Schuttler, R. *et al.* (1980) Longitudinal studies of schizophrenic patients. *Schizophrenia Bulletin*, **6**, 592-605.

Humbert, M., Salvador, L., Segui, J., *et al.* (1986). Estudio interfiabilidad versión española evaluación de sintomas positivos y negativos. *Revista Departmento Psiquiatria*. Facultad de Medicina, University of Barcelona, **13**, 28-36.

Hyde, C.E. (1989). The Manchester scale: A standardised psychiatric assessment for rating chronic psychotic patients. *British Journal of Psychiatry*, **155** (supplement 7), 45.

Iager, A-C., Kirch, D.G. and Wyatt, R.J. (1985). A negative symptom rating scale. *Psychiatry Research*, **16**, 27-36.

Jablensky, A., Schwarz, R. and Tomov, T. (1980). WHO collaborative study on impairment and disabilities associated with schizophrenic disorders. A preliminary communication: Objectives and methods. *Acta Psychiatrica Scandinavica*, **62** (supplement 285), 152-163.

Jackson, H.J., Burgess, P.M., Minas, I.H. and Joshua, S.D. (1990). Psychometric properties of the Manchester Scale. *Acta Psychiatrica Scandinavica*, **81**, 108-113.

Jaeger, J., Bitter, I., Czobor, P. and Volavka, J. (1990). The measurement of subjective experience in schizophrenia: the subjective deficit syndrome scale. *Comprehensive Psychiatry*, **31**, 216-226.

Johnstone, E.C. (1989). The assessment of negative and positive features in schizophrenia. *British Journal of Psychiatry*, **155** (supplement 7), 41-44.

Johnstone, E.C., Owens, D.G.C., Frith, C.D. and Crow, T.J. (1986). The relative stability of positive and negative features in chronic schizophrenia. *British Journal of Psychiatry*, **150**, 60-64.

Johnstone, E.C., Crow, T.J., Frith, C.D., Carney, M.W. and Price, J.S. (1978*a*) Mechanism of the antipsychotic effect in the treatment of acute schizophrenia. *Lancet*, **i**, 848-851.

Johnstone, E.C., Crow, T.J., Frith, C.D., Stevens, M., Kreel, L. and Husband, J. (1978*b*). The dementia of dementia praecox. *Acta Psychiatrica Scandinavia*, **57**, 305-324.

Kay, S.R. (1991). "Positive and Negative Syndromes in Schizophrenia: Assessment and Research". Brunner/Mazel, New York.

Kay, S.R. and Opler, L.A. (1987). The positive-negative dimension in schizophrenia: its validity and significance. *Psychiatric Developments*, **2**, 79-103.

Kay, S.R., Opler, L.A. and Fiszbein, A. (1986). Significance of positive and negative syndromes in chronic schizophrenia. *British Journal of Psychiatry*, **149**, 439-448.

Kay, S.R., Opler, L.A. and Lindenmayer, J-P. (1988) Reliability and validity of the positive and negative symptom scale for schizophrenics. *Psychiatry Research*, **23**, 99-110.

Kay, S.R., Opler, L.A. and Lindenmayer, J-P. (1989). The positive and negative syndrome scale (PANSS): rationale and standardisation. *British Journal of Psychiatry*, **155** (supplement 7), 59-65.

Kirkpatrick, B., Buchanan, R.W., McKenney, P.D., Alphs, L.D. and Carpenter, W.T. (1989). The schedule for the deficit syndrome: an instrument for research in schizophrenia. *Psychiatry Research,* **30**, 119-123.

Koehler, K. and Sauer, H. (1984). Huber's basic symptoms: Another approach to negative psychopathology in schizophrenia. *Comprehensive Psychiatry*, **25**, 174-182.

Krawiecka, M., Goldberg, D. and Vaughan, M.A. (1977). Standardised psychiatric assessment for rating chronic patients. *Acta Psychiatrica Scandinavica*, **55**, 299-308.

Leach, A.M. (1991). Negative symptoms. *Current Opinion in Psychiatry,* **4**, 18-22.

Liddle, P.F. and Barnes, T.R.E. (1988). The subjective experience of deficits in schizophrenia. *Comprehensive Psychiatry*, **29**, 157-164.

McGlashan, T.H. and Carpenter, W.T. (1976). Postpsychotic depression in schizophrenia. *Archives of General Psychiatry*, **33**, 231-239.

McKenna, P.J., Lund, C.E. and Mortimer, A.M. (1989). Negative symptoms: relationship to other schizophrenic classes. *British Journal of Psychiatry*, **155** (supplement 7), 104-107.

Manchanda, R., Saupe, R. and Hirsch, S.R. (1986). Comparison between the brief psychiatric rating scale and the manchester scale for the rating of schizophrenic symptomatology. *Acta Psychiatrica Scandinavica*, **74**, 563-568.

Manchanda, R., Hirsch, S.R. and Barnes, T.R.E. (1989). A review of rating scales for measuring symptom changes in schizophrenic research. *In* "The Instruments of Psychiatric Research". (Ed. C. Thompson), pp 59-86. John Wiley and Sons, Chichester..

Montgomery, S. and Asberg, M. (1979). A new depression scale designed to be sensitive to change. *British Journal of Psychiatry*, **134**, 382-9.

Mortimer, A., McKenna, P.J., Lund, C.E. and Mannuzza, S. (1989). Rating of negative symptoms using the HEN scale. *British Journal of Psychiatry*, **155** (supplement 7), 89-91.

Moscarelli, M., Maffei, C. and Cesano, B.M. (1987). An international perspective on the assessment of positive and negative symptoms in schizophrenia. *American Journal of Psychiatry,* **144**, 1595-1598.

Newcomer, J.W., Faustman, W.O., Yeh, W. and Csernansky, J.G. (1990). Distinguishing depression and negative symptoms in unmedicated patients with schizophrenia. *Psychiatry Research*, **31**, 243-250.

Ohta, T., Okazaki, Y. and Anzai, N. (1984). Reliability of the Japanese version of the scale for the assessment of negative symptoms (SANS). *Japanese Journal of Psychiatry,* **13**, 999-1010

Overall, J.E. (1974). The Brief Psychiatric Rating Scale in psychopharmacology research. *In* "Psychological Measurements in Psychopharmacology: Modern Problems in Pharmacopsychiatry". Vol. 7. (Ed. P. Pichot). pp 67-78. Karger, Basel.

Overall, J.E. and Gorham, D. (1962). The Brief Psychiatric Rating Scale. *Psychological Reports*, **10**, 799-812.

Owens, D.G.C. and Johnstone, E.C. (1980). The disabilities of chronic schizophrenia. Their nature and the factors contributing to their development. *British Journal of Psychiatry*, **136**, 384-395.

Petho, B. and Bitter, I. (1985). Types of complaints in psychiatric and internal medical patients. *Psychopathology*, **18**, 241-253.

Pogue-Geile, M.F. and Harrow, M. (1984). Negative and positive symptoms in schizophrenia and depression: A follow-up. *Schizophrenia Bulletin*, **10**, 371-387.

Pogue-Geile, M.F. and Harrow, M. (1985). Negative symptoms in schizophrenia: their longitudinal course and prognostic importance. *Schizophrenia Bulletin*, **11**, 427-439.

Pogue-Geile, M.F. and Zubin, J. (1988). Negative symptomatology and schizophrenia: a conceptual and empirical review. *International Journal of Mental Health*, **16**, 3-45.

Prosser, E.S., Csernansky, J.G., Kaplan, J., Thiemann, S., Becker, T.J. and Hollister, L.E. (1987). Depression, parkinsonian symptoms, and negative symptoms in schizophrenics treated with neuroleptics. *Journal of Nervous and Mental Disease*, **175**, 100-105.

Reid, W.H., Moore, S.L. and Zimmer, M. (1982). Assessment of affect in schizophrenia. *Journal of Nervous and Mental Disease*, **170**, 266-269.

Roth, M. (1989). Commentary on the contributions of Professor H. Sass, Dr G. Gross and Dr Ch. Mundt *et al.* on "negative" and "basic" symptoms of schizophrenia. *British Journal of Psychiatry*, **155** (supplement 7), 37-40.

Siris, S.G., Adan, F., Cohen, M., Mandeli, J., Aronson, A. and Casey, E. (1988). Post-psychotic depression and negative symptoms: an investigation of syndromal overlap. *American Journal of Psychiatry*, **145**, 1532-1537.

Stern, M.J., Pillsbury, J.A. and Sonnenberg, S.M. (1972). Postpsychotic depression in schizophrenics. *Comprehensive Psychiatry*, **13**, 519-598.

Strauss, J., Carpenter, W.T. and Bartko, J. (1974). The diagnosis and understanding of schizophrenia: Part III. Speculations on the processes that underlie schizophrenic symptoms and signs. *Schizophrenia Bulletin*, **1**, 61-69.

Sommers, A.S. (1985). "Negative symptoms": conceptual and methodological problems. *Schizophrenia Bulletin*, **11**, 364-379.

Thiemann, S., Csernansky, J.G. and Berger, P.A. (1987). Rating scales in research: the case of negative symptoms. *Psychiatry Research*, **20**, 47-55.

Walker, E.F., Harvey, P.D. and Perlman, D. (1988). The positive/negative symptom distinction in psychoses. *Journal of Nervous and Mental Disease*, **176**, 359-363.

Whiteford, H.A., Riney, S.J. and Csernansky, J.G. (1987). Distinguishing depressive and negative symptoms in chronic schizophrenia. *Psychopathology*, **20**, 234-236.

Wykes, T. and Sturt, E. (1986). The measurement of social behaviour in psychiatric patients: an assessment of the reliability and validity of the SBS schedule. *British Journal of Psychiatry*, **148**, 1-11.

6. The Assessment of Affective Symptoms in Schizophrenia

Stuart A. Montgomery, David Baldwin and Deirdre Montgomery

Depressive symptoms occur frequently in patients with a primary diagnosis of schizophrenia. There are a number of reasons why identifying and quantifying the depressive symptoms occurring in schizophrenic patients is important. These include the potential for diagnostic confusion, the bearing that the presence of depressive symptoms may have on prognosis, the effect of antipsychotic medication on the symptoms and the information these symptoms may yield on the nature of the illness.

Prevalence of depressive symptoms in schizophrenia

Estimates of the prevalence of depressive symptoms in patients with schizophrenia vary but even the most conservative suggest that they occur in some 25% of schizophrenic patients suffering an acute episode and other observers have suggested they are present in at least 60% of patients (Donlon *et al.*, 1976; Montgomery, 1979; Knights and Hirsch, 1981). Depressive symptoms are also present in chronic schizophrenia. Barnes *et al.* (1989) reported, for example, that 13% of chronic hospitalized schizophrenic patients complained of depressed mood, with symptoms reaching a full depressive syndrome, and other studies have found higher rates (Planansky and Johnson, 1978).

The depressive symptoms may persist in the absence of overt schizophrenic psychopathology as follow up studies have shown (Falloon *et al.*, 1978; McGlashan and Carpenter, 1976; Mandel *et al.*, 1982). As many as 50% of chronic schizophrenics may report depressive symptoms when followed up after discharge from hospital (Falloon *et al.*, 1978). The depressive symptoms are however particularly associated with acute episodes or exacerbations (Knights and Hirsch, 1981; Curson *et al.*, 1985).

Diagnosis

The potential for uncertainty of diagnosis is obvious when considering that depressive symptoms occur frequently in schizophrenia and delusions are a feature of some depressions. The delusions occurring in major depressive disorder are effectively separated from schizophrenia using the concept of mood congruence though the separation is not always an easy one.

The view that in clearcut schizophrenia depressive symptoms are core features of the schizophrenia is supported by the presence of depressive symptoms in more than half of first episode cases (Johnson, 1981). However, the absence of depressive symptoms in a substantial proportion of schizophrenic patients with marked psychotic features has led other investigators to conclude that they are not core features of schizophrenia.

There remains a group where both schizophrenic and affective symptoms are prominent in whom diagnosis is not straightforward. Schizoaffective disorder, a concept that has had a variety of definitions, is sometimes used to categorize these patients (see also Chapter 1, pages 3 and 5). The relative preponderance of schizophrenic or depressive symptoms in a particular episode does not appear of itself to be of clear predictive value for diagnosis. However, the separate assessment of the depressive symptoms is important since a poorer outcome is reported if in the history there have been episodes of schizophrenic symptoms in the absence of depressive symptoms.

Which Symptoms

Patients suffering from schizophrenia who have clear depressive psychopathology appear in many cases to have the full range of symptoms that would categorize major depression. This has been reported in studies that assessed the depressive symptoms using the Present State Examination interview (Wing *et al.*, 1974). Knights and Hirsch, (1981), Curson *et al.* (1985), Mandel *et al.* (1982) and Barnes *et al.* (1989) reported a similar phenomenon using the Hamilton Rating Scale for depression. The symptoms were specifically examined in one study (Montgomery, 1979) which assessed a sample of 50 schizophrenic patients suffering an acute episode using the Montgomery and Asberg Depression Rating Scale (MADRS) (Montgomery and Asberg, 1979) and the Montgomery Schizophrenia Scale (MSS) (Montgomery *et al.*, 1978), a 12 item scale derived from the Comprehensive Psychopathological Rating Scale (CPRS) (Asberg *et al.*, 1978). The items of the MADRS, which focuses on the core symptoms of depression are reported sadness, apparent sadness, inner tension, reduced sleep, reduced appetite, inability to feel, pessimistic thoughts, lassitude, concentration difficulties, suicidal thoughts. In this sample of patients suffering from schizophrenia depressive symptoms were frequent. All the items of the MADRS were scored in more than 40% of the sample; the mean frequency of occurrence of the 10 items was 61%.

Prognostic value of depressive symptoms

Opinions have varied as to whether the presence of depressive symptoms in clearly diagnosed schizophrenia predicts a better outcome. Earlier studies suggested this might be the case (Vaillant, 1964) but more recent research has not found depressive symptoms to have significant prognostic value (Brockington *et al.*, 1980; Gift *et al.*, 1980). It is however reported that patients suffering from schizophrenia who have depressive symptoms have a higher risk of suicide (Roy, 1986; Prasad, 1986) though studies have not found that depressive symptoms predicted suicide attempts (Allebeck, 1987). Nevertheless the identification of depressive symptoms may have important implications for management.

It is increasingly recognized that depressive symptoms are features of the prodromal phase in first episode illness and predictors of incipient relapse in patients with established schizophrenia (Herz and Melville, 1980). Frequently reported symptoms prior to a relapse are inner tension, reduced appetite, sleep disturbance, poor concentration, lack of interest and depressed mood and these can be recognized by some 70% of schizophrenic patients and more than 90% of their relatives (Herz and Melville, 1980). Since these symptoms may be present for some time before psychotic phenomena appear they may serve as valuable prompts of the need to review medication, and the occurrence of marked affective symptoms in patients with established schizophrenia justifies early intervention with neuroleptic medication (Jolley *et al.*, 1989).

Depressive symptoms and side-effects of drugs
It is important to have a sensitive measure of the depressive symptoms because some investigators have suggested that antipsychotic drugs may have a direct causal role in producing depression (de Alarcon and Carney, 1969; Ananth and Ghadirian, 1980). There is some evidence from placebo-controlled studies to support this, for example Galdi (1983) reported that patients with a genetic loading for schizophrenia and depression were more depressed following neuroleptic medication compared with matched controls.

Disentangling depressive symptoms from drug effects can be a problem since some side-effects, for example some parkinsonian symptoms, are difficult to distinguish from retarded depression. Schizophrenic patients with depressive symptoms may appear wooden in expression, retarded in movement, hypersomnic, disinclined to speak, emotionally withdrawn, lacking in initiative, etc. Rifkin *et al.* (1975) have noted that all of these features may be found in neuroleptic-induced akinesia. Similarly, patients with Parkinson's disease may demonstrate anergia, retardation, anhedonia, depression and bradyphrenia. Similar clinical syndromes may therefore be demonstrated in differing patient groups experiencing dopamine depletion. One solution to the difficulty of distinguishing between symptoms that make up a syndrome and side-effects of drugs that mimic symptoms is to rate the symptoms regardless of possible cause and to record the likely causes.

Depressive symptoms and negative symptoms
One of the most important difficulties in assessing depressive symptoms in schizophrenia is the similarity between certain negative symptoms considered characteristic of schizophrenia and depressive symptoms. The situation is not helped by a certain ambiguity in the scales that measure negative symptoms as to which are the relevant items. The widely used negative symptom scales, for example the Scale for the Assessment of Negative Symptoms (SANS) (Andreasen, 1982) and Positive and Negative Symptom Scale (PANSS) (Kay *et al.*, 1989) differ considerably in their content though they share certain cardinal items such as flatness of affect and poverty of speech. Even if there were agreement on the most important items the problem of distinguishing between negative symptoms and depressive symptoms would remain.

There is some specific overlap between features which characterize negative schizophrenia and depression. Anhedonia, anergia, social withdrawal and poverty of speech are included in scales to measure negative symptoms in schizophrenia and are also all characteristic of depression. Similarly items included on depression rating scales, for example lassitude, inability to feel and concentration difficulties in the MADRS, may be perceived as negative symptoms in schizophrenia.

However a differentiation can be made between negative symptoms of schizophrenia and depressive symptoms. House *et al.* (1987) demonstrated in a study of schizophrenic patients rated with a variety of instruments including the PSE and Psychological Impairments Rating Scale (Jablensky *et al.*, 1980) that depressive symptoms and signs could be reliably distinguished from akinesia and the clinical poverty of affect syndrome. Similar results were reported from a study that compared scores on different measures of psychotic and depressive symptomatology in schizophrenic patients stratified according to predominant positive, negative or mixed symptomatology (Kulhara *et al.*, 1989). Barnes *et al.* (1989) reported that negative features were approximately evenly distributed between depressed and non-depressed schizophrenic patients again suggesting that the two types of symptoms are different and can be distinguished.

Response of depressive symptoms

There is some evidence to suggest that an apparent worsening may occur in the depressive symptoms as the psychotic symptoms, present throughout the episode of illness but only detected after suppression of the psychotic symptoms, appear to be unmasked during treatment. Sensitive measures are needed to detect the appearance of depressive symptoms as well as improvement during treatment. Over time the depressive symptoms appear to improve during successful treatment with antipsychotic medication in parallel with the improvement in psychotic phenomena (Donlon *et al.*, 1976; Knights and Hirsch, 1981) though the response may be a little slower so that there are residual depressive symptoms after the response of the psychotic symptoms.

Choice of scales to measure depressive symptoms in schizophrenia

There have been rather few attempts to determine how reliably the depressive symptoms occurring in schizophrenia can be measured. There are features of the illness that are likely to reduce the overall and the expected test retest reliabilities, for example lack of insight and poverty of affect (Strian *et al.*, 1981; Donlon *et al.*, 1976).

There are no scales developed specifically to assess depressive symptoms in schizophrenia and most studies that have addressed the problem have therefore used scales developed for another purpose. For example the Hamilton Rating Scale for Depression (Hamilton, 1960) was used by Craig *et al.* (1985) in a comparison with the Brief Psychiatric Rating Scale (Overall and Gorham, 1962) and the Affective Flattening Scale (Andreasen, 1979). The use of scale developed specifically for use in depression to measure symptoms in schizophrenia may be considered a doubtful approach. The view has been put forward that the affective psychopathology found in schizophrenic patients is qualitatively different to that exhibited in patients suffering from primary affective disorders (van Putten and May, 1978; Mandel *et al.*, 1982) and the use of traditional depression rating scales may not therefore be appropriate.

Nevertheless it does appear to be possible to measure the depressive symptoms as a number of studies that have compared rating scales have shown. The study of Craig *et al.* (1985) found that there was an acceptable degree of agreement between the overall scores on the scales used to measure depressive and psychotic symptoms though a number of the items were inconsistently rated. These items tended to reflect psychological and somatic symptoms: by contrast, items measuring agitation, retardation and psychosis showed high levels of interscale reliability. How accurate or useful the measures are will depend on the type of scale.

If conventional depression rating scales can be used in schizophrenic patients the choice of which one will depend on the sensitivity, reliability and the robustness of the scale.

The Assessment Procedures

Self Rating Scales

Beck Depression Inventory
(Beck, 1961)

Zung self-rating depression scale
(Zung, 1956)

Utility
Although self rating scales have been used for comparative purposes in groups of schizophrenic patients, their use is limited and is not recommended. It is no surprise that correlations between self-reported and observer-rated measures of depression in schizophrenia have been found to be low (Craig and van Natta, 1976; Strian *et al.*, 1981). Self rating scales are limited by the need for a certain level of motivation, concentration, and education, as well as insight on the part of the patient required to fill them in. Numerous studies have also shown that self rating scales provide a less sensitive measure of change in severity than observer rating scales because of the increased variability associated with their use. Although it is reported that a substantial proportion of schizophrenic patients can recognize depressive symptoms in themselves prior to a relapse there is an important difference between identifying presence or absence of a symptom and giving an accurate measure of severity.

Observer Rating Scales

The choice of an observer rating scale is made from three general categories: general scales of psychopathology that include both schizophrenic items and depressive items, specific schizophrenia scales that include one or more depressive items, and scales developed specifically for use in depressive illness.

General Scales

Present State Examination (PSE)
(Wing et al., 1974) (see also Chapter 1)

This scale was developed as a diagnostic instrument to cover the range of psychiatric illness. Patients with no symptoms or who are able to give clear answers would be rapidly rated with the 54 obligatory questions but the supplementary questions make this a long instrument which would entail a lengthy interview with many patients suffering from schizophrenia.

If symptoms are present they are scored in categories of either moderate or severe. The rater must be fully trained and familiar with the glossary provided for rating the items. Depressive items are included: depressed mood, hopelessness, suicidal plans, social withdrawal, inferiority feelings, guilt, disturbance in appetite, disturbance in sleep, retardation are all questioned as are somatic and psychic anxiety and concentration difficulties.

Reliability and validity
The scale was extensively tested in development and the results published and has been used very widely as a diagnostic instrument.

Utility
This is a diagnostic instrument and is based on diagnostic hierarchical principles. There is a major drawback in using this type of approach for rating depressive symptoms in schizophrenia because of the tendency for the questions to lead to a diagnosis and the risk of underestimating apparently secondary features. For the purpose of diagnosis the presence or absence of symptoms is the critical factor but if a scale is being selected for use in assessing the severity of symptoms and possible change with treatment, greater sensitivity and range of assessment are needed. Although scales developed for diagnostic and classificatory purposes have been used to measure severity and change in general, it is inappropriate to use scales for purposes other than that for which they were designed.

Comprehensive Psychopathological Rating Scale (CPRS)
(Asberg et al., 1978) (see also Chapters 2 and 3)

The Comprehensive Psychopathological Rating Scale was developed to record the severity of psychopathology in the range of psychiatric illness. Unlike most earlier scales it was constructed explicitly to measure change in psychopathology and the items that were thought most likely to change with treatment were included.

The rating time will vary with the type of patient and the diagnosis and also on whether the full list of items is used. A guide time of 1 hour for an initial interview is given though this is likely to be considerably shorter with many patients.

The scale is a pool of 65 items from which subscales for specific syndromes can be constructed. Forty of the items are rated on the basis of what the patient reports and 23 on the basis of observation, two further items provide a global impression of severity and of the reliability of the rating. The ratings are based on all the information gathered from an interview which follows as closely as possible the clinical psychiatric interview. This technique is considered a more appropriate way of obtaining a valid rating than the use of a structured interview schedule. The rating period is likely to be most commonly a week but the scale can also be used for shorter or longer rating periods.

Each item is scored from 0 (normal functioning) to 3 (extreme degree of symptom). The points 0, 1, 2, 3 have defined severity levels which form part of the scale and the rater is expected to use the half points between these peg points as well, creating a 7 point scale. The CPRS includes the full range of depressive symptoms described more fully below.

Reliability and validity
Inter-rater reliabilities for different sections of the total item pool are published, as are crosscultural reliabilities (Montgomery et al., 1978). Normative data are not published. The scale is in wide use in different patient groups in treatment studies using the main subpools of the items that have been published.

Utility
The approach taken in developing the CPRS was that psychopathology should be recorded irrespective of the rater's view on cause or meaning and has the advantage that assessments are made without the bias of theoretical standpoints on aetiology. This allows a more objective assessment of psychopathology. The preamble to the scale suggests that raters should be experienced and trained in rating but it has been shown in practice that good inter-rater reliabilities are obtained with a small amount of training and the scale is readily handled by both medical and related disciplines (Montgomery et al., 1978).

Schedule for Affective Disorders and Schizophrenia (SADS)
(Endicott and Spitzer, 1978) (see also Chapter 4)

Following the development of this scale, which was intended for diagnostic purposes, a supplementary version to measure change was constructed. Since the full range of psychopathology in affective disorders and schizophrenia is covered it can be used to measure depressive symptoms in schizophrenia. The items are scored on a 6 or 7 point scale and defined severity levels are specified.

Utility
The scale is intended to be sufficiently comprehensive to be used in the different clinical syndromes so that the full range of depressive symptomatology is covered. The authors have reported a study showing that a reliable Hamilton Depression Rating Scale score can be extracted from the scores recorded on the SADS in

depressed patients. How adequately the depressive symptoms in schizophrenic patients are scored is not reported. In practice the scale may be seen as a group of separate scales covering different illnesses.

Schizophrenia Scales

Brief Psychiatric Rating Scale (BPRS)
(Overall and Gorham, 1962) (see also Chapters 2, 3 and 5)

The Brief Psychiatric Rating Scale is used primarily for assessing psychotic illness. The length of the interview will vary to some extent according to the severity of the illness and the ability of the patient to respond to the questions, but will take in the order of 15-30 minutes.

The items are rated on a 7 point scale from not present to extremely severe and a glossary is provided to give a framework for the rating. Depressive items include depressive mood under which degree or despondency is rated without inference from retardation, etc., and guilt feelings. Subjective anxiety is also rated.

Utility
The scale includes both symptoms for measuring psychosis and depressive items in one instrument. However it is limited since it does not cover the range of depressive symptomatology that is likely to occur in schizophrenia. Difficulty is often experienced in making a distinction between emotional withdrawal, blunted affect, retardation and depressive mood and the rater may not find it easy where to put the emphasis of rating.

Despite its widely acknowledged shortcomings the BPRS has been one of the most extensively used scales in studies of schizophrenia and therefore has the advantage of familiarity. However, although drug placebo differences have been demonstrated using the scale, it is generally thought to be relatively insensitive to change (for example Montgomery, 1979 and 1992).

Montgomery Schizophrenia Scale (MSS)
(Montgomery et al., 1978) (see also Chapters 2 and 3)

This scale was developed with the specific objective of being sensitive to treatment change in patients already diagnosed as suffering from schizophrenia. It covers schizophrenic symptomatology but also includes three depressive items. The scale was constructed from items drawn from the CPRS (Asberg *et al.*, 1978) which were selected on the basis of frequency of occurrence and demonstrated sensitivity to change.

It is a short scale, 12 items, and the rating represents clinical judgement made on the basis of an adequate interview covering the whole range of phenomena experienced by schizophrenic patients in sufficient detail for a rating of individual items to be made. The severity, the frequency and the duration of the phenomena all contribute to the rating. Items are scored on a 7 point scale, 0 normal to 6 very severe. Operational severity definitions are provided for the points 0, 2, 4, and 6 with undefined intervening scores for patients who fall between two levels of defined severity.

Reliability and validity
This scale is not a diagnostic scale but was designed as a measure of severity in patients already diagnosed as schizophrenic. Its improved sensitivity to treatment change has been demonstrated in comparison to the BPS (Montgomery *et al.*, 1978*c*). Good inter-rater reliabilities are reported both on the individual items and the total scale (Montgomery *et al.*, 1978*c*).

Utility
The scale is short and designed for ratings to be made working from the text with the item definitions. The items were only selected if they both occurred frequently and were sensitive to change. Three of the items that reach these criteria are depressive and occur in the Montgomery and Asberg Depression Rating Scale (Montgomery and Asberg, 1979). These are Reported Sadness, Pessimistic Thoughts and Inability to Feel, which appear to be sensitive to change in schizophrenia as well as depression. Inability to feel might be thought to be potentially difficult to distinguish from poverty of affect but this feature is rated separately in the MSS on an observed item, Inappropriate Emotion.

Manchester Scale (MS)
(Krawiecka et al., 1977) (see also Chapters 2, 3 and 5)

The scale is designed to assess symptom severity in patients suffering from schizophrenia and covers the range of expected schizophrenic psychopathology. It contains nine items which are rated on a 5 point scale. The scale includes a specific item for depression.

Utility
The MS provides an easily used scale to cover the range of schizophrenic symptoms but its coverage of the depressive symptoms is limited. As a result, a differentiation between such features as blunted affect or retardation and depressive symptomatology is unlikely to be reliable.

Negative Symptom Scales

Scale for the Assessment of Negative Symptoms (SANS)
(Andreasen, 1982) (see also Chapters 5 and 6)

Negative Symptom Rating Scale (NSRS)
(Iager, 1984) (see also Chapter 5)

Positive and Negative Symptom Scale (PANSS)
(Kay, et al., 1989; Kay, 1991) (see also Chapter 5)

Utility

These scales, described more fully in Chapter 5, might be used to measure depressive symptoms but it is unlikely that they would provide sensitive measures. Scales for measuring negative symptoms include items that are depressive in tone rather than addressing the presence of depressive symptoms *per se*. For example the SANS includes a section for anhedonia, the PANSS includes emotional withdrawal and social withdrawal and all the scales cover affective blunting. Negative symptoms scales can thus provide only an indirect and imperfect measure of depressive symptoms.

The set of the rater with such scales is to assess schizophrenic symptoms and the balance between what is a depressive symptom and what is a negative symptom of schizophrenia is very likely to be biased. Because of the risk of interpreting depressive symptoms as the blunted affect characteristic of schizophrenia and vice versa, the use of a scale that specifically measures depressive symptoms is recommended if a negative symptoms scale is used.

Depression Rating Scales

The use of traditional depression rating scales to measure depressive symptoms in schizophrenia is a somewhat problematic enterprise since it involves using scales for purposes for which they were not specifically designed or tested. Nevertheless, the two currently most widely used observer rating scales for depression, the Montgomery and Asberg Depression Rating Scale (MADRS) (Montgomery and Asberg, 1979) and the Hamilton Rating Scale for Depression (Hamilton, 1960) have both been used successfully to measure these symptoms.

Montgomery and Asberg Depression Rating Scale (MADRS)
(Montgomery and Asberg, 1979)

This scale drew on the CPRS (Asberg *et al.*, 1978) to construct a sensitive measure of change in patients diagnosed as suffering from depression. The scale has 10 items which focus on the core symptoms of depression and the length of time required for rating, which is based on the clinical interview, will be relatively short in a patient with moderate depression and good insight. Assessment in schizophrenic patients may take longer. Nine of the items are rated on the patient's report and one on observation of the patient. The items are rated on a 7 point scale, 0 normal to 6 severe. Operational definitions of severity levels are give for 0, 2, 4 and 6, the intermediate points being undefined for patients falling between two levels of severity. The scale is designed so that the rater has the definitions before him or her in making the rating.

Reliability and validity

The total score of all 10 items provides an overall level of severity of depression but the individual items have been constructed for individual analysis. The sensitivity of both the total score and the scores of individual items have been shown to be sensitive to change in conventional depression and in other patient groups with depressive syndromes, for example personality disorders (Montgomery *et al.*, 1983). Validity and reliabilities are reported (Montgomery and Asberg, 1979) and inter-rater reliabilities are good for the individual items and for the total score (Montgomery *et al.*, 1978*b*). Its reliability when used by general practitioners, nurses and psychologists, compared with psychiatrists is also good (Montgomery *et al.*, 1978*a*).

Utility

The advantage of using the MADRS to measure depressive symptoms in schizophrenia is that, although it is not a diagnostic scale and was designed to be sensitive to change in depression, its construction is based on the objective assessment of the reported or observed features. If a patient with schizophrenia manifests depressive symptoms these are rated regardless of cause or what else they might reflect. An accurate measure of the severity of the symptoms can thus be obtained. In some cases there may be overlap between the item inability to feel and affective blunting. The emphasis in the MADRS item is on the depressive aspect of loss of pleasure and separation of the features for rating is relatively straightforward. The other item that may cause similar difficulty is lassitude. In some patient groups with predominant negative symptoms the total MADRS score may not give as accurate measure of severity as it would, for example, in a group of depressed patients. However, the individual items of the scale have been constructed for separate analysis and in negative symptom groups this will provide useful information.

Hamilton Rating Scale for Depression (HRSD)
(Hamilton, 1960)

The scale was based on a series of items thought by Hamilton to be representative of depressive illness and was the most widely used observer rating scale in studies of treatment of depression. It was designed for measuring severity and in the second publication four items were excluded since it appeared that they were diagnostic rather than severity measures.

The 17 item scale covers the range of symptoms expected in a depressed population. The original directions for raters suggested that ratings should be based on the average of the ratings made by two independent raters on the basis of a clinical interview. Although a general glossary is supplied the severity definitions are for the most part not specific. The total score gives the assessment of severity of depression. The individual items are not designed to be separately analyzed but general factors have been derived to look at different aspects of the illness.

Utility

The scale covers the range of depressive symptoms but includes a disproportionate number of anxiety symptoms which often causes problems in assessing patients with depression or anxiety. It may be even more of a problem in schizophrenic patients since the anxiety items in depression scales are not always as sensitive when used in schizophrenic populations (Montgomery *et al.*, 1978*c*). The total score which is normally used to give an assessment of severity of depression may therefore be considerably less sensitive as a measure of change. The scale provides a measure of the depressive symptoms but it is difficult to assess change on individual items because the scale was not designed for this type of analysis.

Conclusions

Depressive symptoms occur frequently in schizophrenia, they change with treatment with antipsychotic medication, and may predict relapse. There is some overlap between symptoms considered depressive and those considered schizophrenic and potential for confusion in assessment. These symptoms should be specifically measured either with a schizophrenia scale that includes a sufficient number of clearly depressive items or with a depression rating scale, preferably one that permits analysis of individual items.

References

Allebeck , P., Varla, A., Kristanjansson, S. and Wistedt, B. (1987). Risk factors for suicide among patients with schizophrenia. *Acta Psychiatrica Scandinavica,* **76**, 414-419.

Ananth, J. and Ghadirian, A.M. (1980). Drug induced mood disorder. *International Pharmacopsychiatry,* **15**, 58-73.

Andreasen, N.C. (1979). Thought, language and communication disorders: I Clinical assessment definition of terms, and evaluation of their reliability. *Archives of General Psychiatry*, **36**, 1315.

Andreasen, N.C. (1981). "The Scale of the Assessment of Negative Symptoms". University of Iowa, Iowa City.

Andreasen, N.C. (1982). Negative symptoms in schizophrenia: definition and reliability. *Archives of General Psychiatry*, **39**, 784.

Asberg, M., Montgomery, S.A., Perris, C., Schalling, D. and Sedvall, G. (1978). The comprehensive psychopathological rating scale. *Acta Psychiatrica Scandinavica,* Suppl. 277, 5-7.

Barnes, T.R.E., Curson, D.A., Liddle, P.F. and Patel, M. (1989). The nature and prevalence of depression in chronic schizophrenic inpatients. *British Journal of Psychiatry*, **154**, 486-491.

Beck, A.T., Ward, C.H., Mendelson, M., Mock, J.E. and Erbaugh, J.K. (1961). An inventory for measuring depression. *Comprehensive Psychiatry Journal*, **2**, 163-170.

Brockington, I.F., Wainwright, S. and Kendell, R.E. (1980). Manic patients with schizophrenia or paranoid symptoms. *Psychological Medicine,* **10**, 73.

Craig, T.J. and van Natta, P.A. (1976). Presence and persistence of depressive symptoms in patient and community populations. *American Journal of Psychiatry,* **133**, 1426-1429.

Craig, T.J., Richardson, M.A., Pass, R. *et al.* (1985). Measurement of mood and affect in schizophrenic inpatients. *American Journal of Psychiatry*, **142**, 1272-1277.

Curson, D.A., Barnes, T.R.E., Bamber, R.W. *et al.* (1985). Long term depot maintenance of chronic schizophrenic outpatients. The seven year follow-up of the Medical Research Council fluphenazine/placebo trial. II, The incidence of compliance problems side-effects, neurotic symptoms and depression. *British Journal of Psychiatry*, **146**, 469-474.

de Alarcon, R. and Carney, M.W.P. (1969). Severe depressive mood changes following slow release intra-muscular fluphenazine injection. *British Medical Journal*, **iii**, 564-567.

Donlon, P.T., Rada, R.T. and Arora, K.K. (1976). Depression and the reintegration phase of acute schizophrenia. *American Journal of Psychiatry*, **133**, 1265-1268.

Endicott, J. and Spitzer, R.L. (1978). A diagnostic interview: the schedule for affective disorders and schizophrenia (SADS). *Archives of General Psychiatry*, **35**, 837.

Falloon, I., Watt, D.C. and Shepherd, M. (1978). A comparative controlled trial of pimozide and fluphenazine diaconate in the continuation therapy of schizophrenia. *Psychological Medicine*, **8**, 59-70.

Galdi, J. (1983). The causality of depression in schizophrenia. *British Journal of Psychiatry*, **142**, 621-624.

Gift, T.E., Strauss, J.S., Kokes, R.F., Harder, D.W. and Ritzler, B.A. (1980). Schizophrenia: affect and outcome. *American Journal of Psychiatry*, **137**, 580-585.

Hamilton, M. (1960). A rating scale for depression. *Journal of Neurology, Neurosurgery and Psychiatry*, **23**, 56-62.

Herz, M.I. and Melville, C. (1980). Relapse in schizophrenia. *American Journal of Psychiatry*, **137**, 801-805.

House, A., Bostocke, J. and Cooper, J. (1987). Depressive syndromes in the year following onset of a first schizophrenic illness. *British Journal of Psychiatry*, **151**, 772-779.

Iager, A.C., Kirch, D.G. and Wyatt, R.J. (1985). A negative symptom rating scale. *Psychiatric Research*, **16**, 27-36.

Jablensky, A., Schwarz, R. and Tomov, T. (1980). WHO collaborative study on impairments and disabilities associated with schizophrenic disorders: a preliminary communication: objectives and methods. *Acta Psychiatrica Scandinavica*, **6**, (Suppl. 285), 152-163.

Johnson, D.A.W. (1981). Studies of depressive symptoms in schizophrenia. The prevalence of depression and its possible cause. *British Journal of Psychiatry*, **139**, 89-101.

Jolley, A.G., Hirsch, S.R., McRink, A. and Manchanda, R. (1989). Trial of brief intermittent neuroleptic prophylaxis for selected schizophrenic outpatients: Clinical outcome at one year followup. *British Medical Journal*, **298**, 985-990.

Kay, S.R. (1991). "Positive and Negative Syndromes in Schizophrenia: Assessment and Research". Brunner/Mazel, New York.

Kay, S.R., Opler, L.A. and Lindenmayer, J.P. (1989). The positive and negative syndrome scale (PANSS): rationale and standardization. *British Journal of Psychiatry*, **155**, (Suppl. 7), 59-65.

Knights, A. and Hirsch, S.R. (1981). "Revealed" depression and drug treatment for schizophrenia. *Archives of General Psychiatry*, **38**, 800-811.

Krawiecka, M., Goldberg, D. and Vaughan, M.A. (1977). Standardised psychiatric assessment for rating chronic patients. *Acta Psychiatrica Scandinavica*, **55**, 299-308.

Kulhara, P., Avasthi, A., Chadda, R., Chandiramani, K., Mattoo, S.K., Kota, S.K. and Joseph, S. (1989). Negative and depressive symptoms in schizophrenia. *British Journal of Psychiatry*, **154**, 207-211.

Mandel, M.R., Severe, J.B., Schooler, N.R. *et al.* (1982). Development and prediction of postpsychotic depression in neuroleptic-treated schizophrenics. *Archives of General Psychiatry*, **39**, 197-203.

McGlashan, T.H. and Carpenter, W.T. (1976*a*). An investigation of the postpsychotic depressive syndrome. *American Journal Psychiatry*, **133**, 14-19.

McGlashan, T.H.and Carpenter, W.T. (1976*b*). Post-Psychotic depression in schizophrenia. *Archives of General Psychiatry*, **33**, 231-239.

Montgomery, S.A. (1979). Depressive symptoms in acute schizophrenia. *Neuro-Psychopharmacology*, **3**, 429-433.

Montgomery, S.A. and Asberg, M. (1979). A new depression scale designed to be sensitive to change. *British Journal of Psychiatry*, **134**, 382-389.

Montgomery, S.A., Asberg, M. Jornstedt, L., Thoren, P., Traskman, L., McAuley, R., Montgomery, D. and Shaw, P. (1978*a*). Reliability of the CPRS between the disciplines of psychiatry, general practice, nursing, and psychology in depressed patients. *Acta Psychiatrica Scandinavica*, **271**, 29-32.

Montgomery, S.A., Asberg, M., Traskman, L. and Montgomery, D. (1978*b*). Cross cultural studies on the use of the CPRS in English and Swedish depressed patients. *Acta Psychiatrica Scandinavica*, **86**, (Suppl. 2), 97-130.

Montgomery, S.A., Taylor, P. and Montgomery, D. (1978*c*). Development of a schizophrenia scale sensitive to change. *Neuropharmacology*, **17**, 1053-1071.

Montgomery, S.A., Roy, D. and Montgomery, D. (1983). The prevention of recurrent suicidal acts. *British Journal of Clinical Pharmacology*, **15**, 183S-188S.

Montgomery, S.A., Green, M., Rimon, R. *et al.* (1992). Inadequate treatment response to des-enkephalin-γ-endorphin compared with thioridazine and placebo in schizophrenia. *Acta Psychiatrica Scandinavica*, **86**, 97-103.

Overall, J.E. and Gorham, D.R. (1962). The brief psychiatric rating scale. *Psychological Reports*, **10**, 799-812.

Planansky, K. and Johnson, R. (1978). Depressive syndromes in schizophrenia. *Acta Psychiatrica Scandinavica*, **57**, 207-218.

Prasad, A.J. (1986). Attempted suicide in hospitalized schizophrenics. *Acta Psychiatrica Scandinavica*, **74**, 41-42.

Rifkin, A., Quitkin, F. and Klein, S.F. (1975). Akinesia, a poorly recognized drug-induced extrapyramidal behaviour disorder. *Archives of General Psychiatry*, **32**, 672-674.

Roy, A. (1986). Depression, attempted suicide, and suicide in patients with chronic schizophrenia. *Psychiatric Clinics of North America*, **9**, 193-206.

Strian, F., Heger, R. and Klicpera, C. (1981). The course of depression for different types of schizophrenia. *Psychiatry Clinics*, (*Basel*) **14**, 205-214.

Vaillant, G.E. (1964). Prospective prediction of schizophrenic remission. *Archives of General Psychiatry*, **11**, 509.

van Putten, T. and May, P.R.A. (1978). Akinetic depression in schizophrenia. *Archives of General Psychiatry*, **35**, 1101-1107.

Wing, J.K., Cooper, J.E. and Sartorius, N. (1974). "The Measurement and Classification of Psychiatric Symptoms". Cambridge University Press, London.

Zung, W.W.K. (1965). A self-rating depression scale. *Archives of General Psychiatry*, **12**, 63-70.

7. The Assessment of Cognitive Functioning in Clinical Practice

Hazel E. Nelson

Unlike many other assessment procedures for the psychoses, assessment of cognitive functioning in clinical practice is not undertaken to describe and measure psychotic phenomena, or to assist in diagnosis. Despite extensive and detailed investigations over the years, psychologists have been unable to define a distinctive pattern of cognitive deficits associated with schizophrenia which could be used as a diagnostic indicator. Intellectual deterioration is not uncommon in schizophrenia: when it occurs it is indistinguishable on standard neuropsychological test batteries from intellectual deterioration that results from diffuse brain damage (see Goldstein, 1986, for review). The presence and extent of intellectual deterioration in schizophrenic subjects has been related to structural changes in the brain that are similar to those seen in patients with dementing disorders (Bilder et al., 1988). There is usually a decrease in level of intellectual functioning after onset of illness but it is not clear whether intellectual decline is progressive. Several studies suggest that there may be a modest improvement with improvement in psychotic symptomatology, though chronic schizophrenics generally continue to score in the brain damaged range on neuropsychological tests (see Heaton and Crowley, 1981, for review).

Studies have generally reported that chronic patients perform more poorly than acute patients on cognitive tests (e.g. Shapiro and Nelson, 1955) but to some extent this may reflect biased sampling. Chronic patients are often drawn from a hospital population but they will not be a representative sample of all chronic patients, most of whom manage to live in the community: in particular, they will probably not be a representative sample with respect to intellectual status since intellectual status may be one important factor in determining whether chronic psychiatric patients end up in long-stay hospital care or in the community (Johnstone et al., 1981).

The Process of Assessment

Patients are sometimes suspicious of "psychology" or "tests" so it should be explained at the outset that the questions to be asked will be straightforward, with no catches or hidden meanings. It should also be explained that some of the tests will be made harder and harder until errors are made, and that such errors are normal and must be expected.

One of the major problems in assessing psychotic patients, especially the more chronically ill, is their low tolerance of the formal test situation. If a patient refuses to go for formal assessment, a more informal approach on his own territory may be successful, although this will inevitably limit the scope of the results that can be obtained. More commonly, patients will agree to testing but will remain for only a short period. Patients may find the prolonged one-to-one social situation aversive, and it may be necessary to keep sessions short. The session should be finished whilst the patient is still co-operative enough to agree to further testing at another time: if the session is terminated by the patient walking out it is far less likely that he will be persuaded to attend another session in the future.

Where the patient's tolerance of testing may be limited, it is advisable to administer the most important tests first, so that some meaningful results will have been obtained even if the assessment cannot be completed. Individual tests or sub-tests should always be completed at one sitting since there may be short term practice or interference effects from early to late items. Strictly speaking, batteries of tests such as the WAIS-R should also be completed at one sitting since this is how they were standardized. In practice, however, the results obtained from psychotic subjects will probably provide a more valid measure of functioning if they are completed in more than one session by a subject who is co-operative and attentive than if they are completed in a single session by a subject who becomes distracted and unco-operative.

The large majority of patients will co-operate if the tasks are simple enough, suggesting that their intolerance of testing is actually an intolerance for questions that are too difficult and an intolerance for frequent failure. Most cognitive tests assess functioning across the whole normal range and are constructed either so that testing with increasingly difficult items continues until a certain number of errors have been made, or so that some errors are made by even the brightest subjects. Inevitably, these tests are experienced as difficult by the less able psychotic patients and "failures" may come more frequently than "successes". In contrast, tests that are designed specifically to detect deficits rather than measure across the whole normal range may require only one or two errors to indicate abnormality. Patients experience these latter tests as easy and will probably feel satisfied with their test performance even when obtaining an abnormally poor score. In order to maintain co-operation, tests which appear to the subject to be easy should be administered before the more difficult ones, given the proviso that the more important tests precede the less important ones.

The test results obtained during an assessment give a valid estimate of the patient's level of functioning at that particular time and in that particular place, but in order to estimate his " potential" level of functioning, which is generally taken to mean his level of functioning when his psychotic symptoms have been brought under the best possible control, one must estimate how much his performance might improve if this latter state were to be achieved. This is not an easy estimate to make, even for an experienced clinician, and the approximate nature of these estimates should always be made clear in reports.

Poor motivation and distractability are common features of a psychotic disturbance and, when present, will undoubtedly affect the results obtained in a formal assessment. Tests requiring more prolonged concentration and effort will tend to be more severely affected, so that difficult or long items tend to be particularly susceptible to these effects. Items which give bonus points for speed also tend to be disproportionately affected. If present, thought disorder will adversely affect test results. Responses to easier items may be surprisingly lucid and to the point, but the thought disorder will become more evident on questions that the subject finds difficult.

Most psychotic patients referred for cognitive assessment will be receiving medication; the effect of this on the test results will depend not only on the particular drug and dosage that the patient is receiving (see Heaton and Crowley, 1981, for review) but also on the effect that this has on his psychotic symptoms. Studies with non-psychiatric populations have suggested that neuroleptics with anticholinergic effects may adversely affect cognitive test results, as may drugs with a high sedative effect, but it is not clear whether these drugs similarly affect psychotic subjects. In general, psychotic subjects seem to have a greater tolerance for the effects of high doses of neuroleptic drugs than non-psychotic subjects, so it may be that the adverse effect on cognitive tests is correspondingly less. The evidence reviewed by Heaton and Crowley (1981) suggests that stable levels of neuroleptic medication do not adversely affect performance on cognitive tasks, if anything scores may be improved slightly due to improved attention and concentration, but in view of the uncertainty about the short-term side-effects of these drugs it is recommended that cognitive assessment should not be undertaken within a couple of weeks of a major change in medication.

When a test is readministered a change in test score may occur as the result of errors within the test itself (all cognitive tests are subject to test error to some degree) or practice effect, as well as a change in the function being assessed. The significance of a change in test score, that is the probability that it reflects a true change in the function being assessed rather than test error or practice effects, can be calculated if the appropriate reliability data is available (Payne and Gwynne-Jones, 1957). In the absence of appropriate test/retest data the assessor will have to use his experience to gauge how long should be left between retests to minimize practice effects, some tests being much more susceptible to practice effects than others. Practice effects may also depend to some extent on characteristics of the subjects concerned, in particular less motivated subjects will tend to concentrate less and spend less time trying to solve difficult items and so have less opportunity for learning. Subjects who substantially underachieve on the first occasion may also be less affected by practice effects if this underachievement means less exposure to the harder items reached on the second occasion.

If parallel forms of a test are available these should be used for retesting over short periods but retesting with different material will introduce another possible source of error when assessing changes in levels of functioning. When retesting over longer periods, it is probably more reliable to retest with the same test rather than with a parallel form because the effects of practice will be less than the effects of using different test materials.

When reassessing a subject it is important to bear in mind the possibility that prior exposure to the test may have subtly changed the nature of the test in the retest situation. This is particularly likely to occur if an element of the test is its novelty or uncertainty, as for example in the Wisconsin Card Sorting Test (Berg, 1948), or if the test instructions are unintentionally vague. Test instruction should be made as explicit as possible to ensure that the test/retest situations are comparable with respect to the subject's expectations and knowledge of test requirements.

The Assessment Procedures

Assessment of Eyesight

Before proceeding with tests using visual material the assessor should check that the subject's visual acuity is sufficient for the material concerned. Poor visual acuity, especially amongst more elderly chronic patients, is not a trivial problem. For example, in a recent study of chronic schizophrenic inpatients (Nelson *et al.*, 1990) 21% were found to have no glasses and poor eyesight such that they would have been unable to read this text.

Reading Test Types
(Keeler Ltd.)

The Reading Test Types consist of short passages of different sized print, sections of which the subject reads aloud to determine the smallest size of print that he can distinguish. It takes less than a minute to administer. If the subject is unable to read text then individual letters can be used.

A pilot study undertaken recently at our hospital indicated that scores on the performance scale of the WAIS-R are not adversely affected by poor eyesight in subjects who can read at least size N8 print from the reading test types. The possible effects of poor eyesight on other tests depend on the size and detail of the test materials used.

Utility
This test is so quick and easy to administer that it should be given routinely before all formal assessments.

Assessment of Current Level of Intellectual Functioning

A common reason for referring a psychotic patient for cognitive assessment is to determine his general level of intellectual functioning in order to set the most appropriate goals for rehabilitation and to develop a rehabilitation programme that is within his capabilities.

Current level of intellectual functioning may also have implications for the type of therapy attempted and how it is conducted. For example, many of the cognitive therapies rely on the use of rational argument and deductions and so may be inappropriate or have to be significantly modified for a patient of low intelligence. The psychodynamic therapies may also have to be modified according to the patient's ability to understand and communicate. Behaviour therapies tend to be less affected by low intelligence but even so progress is generally better if the patient understands and actively co-operates in his programme, and of course for ethical reasons he should be capable of understanding his programme and its implications before agreeing to take part in it.

Assessment and reassessment may be used to measure the effects of a drug treatment or some other type of intervention on the cognitive functioning of a psychotic patient. There may be interest in one particular aspect of cognition, such as memory, or it may be the effect on general intellectual level that is of interest. Whatever the cognitive function being assessed, it is the measure of change that is important in this case rather than the measure of level relative to the normal population.

Wechsler Adult Intelligence Scale – Revised (WAIS-R)
(Wechsler, 1981)

The WAIS-R comprises 11 subtests, six in the verbal scale and five in the performance scale, which tap a wide range of cognitive functioning. From these scores a Verbal IQ, a Performance (non-verbal) IQ and a Full-Scale IQ can be computed. The complete scale normally takes about one and a half hours to administer, but it can take considerably longer with distractable patients.

The assessor and subject interact throughout the assessment so the test has to be administered on an individual basis. All subtests bar one have items of graded difficulty and testing with each subtest continues until a certain number of errors are made or until the last item is reached. Some subtests have time limits for each question and in some subtests bonus points are awarded for speed.

The raw score for each subtest is converted into a scaled score, which is not age-corrected, and into an age-scaled score, which is corrected for age effects. These scaled scores have a mean of 10 and a standard deviation of 3. The subtest scaled scores in the Verbal and Performance scales are summed, and reference to IQ tables are provided for different age ranges between 16 and 75 years, so WAIS-R IQs are corrected for ageing effects. Within the normal population, WAIS-R IQs have a mean of 100 and a standard deviation of 15, i.e. 66% of the normal population have IQs between 85 and 115 and 96% of the population have IQs between 70 and 130.

Reliability and validity

The WAIS-R was standardized on 1880 people in the United States of America, who were selected so as to provide a representative sample of the total population with respect to age, sex, race, education and occupation.

The test manual reports split half or test/re-test reliabilities for individual subtests ranging from 0.52 to 0.96, but most fall in the 0.8 decile. Split half reliability coefficients for the IQs are higher, in the 0.9 decile.

The validity of the WAIS (of which the WAIS-R is a revised and updated version) as a measure of general intelligence has been established in a large number of studies that have looked at the relationship between IQ scores and factors such as academic success and occupational achievement (see Matarazzo, 1972, for review) and the relationship between WAIS IQs and other tests of intelligence (see Zimmerman and Woo-Sam, 1973, for review). Factor analytic studies (e.g. Canavan *et al.*, 1986) have confirmed the validity of the WAIS-R as a measure of general intelligence. A verbal-general IQ and a spatial-performance IQ can be calculated from Canavan *et al.*'s rotated factor solution of the WAIS-R inter-correlation matrix. These approximate to the Verbal and Performance IQs respectively, but are factorially purer measures and should be preferred for indicating left/right hemisphere differences.

Utility

The WAIS-R incorporates two major aspects of intelligence, the ability to use previously acquired knowledge and the ability to solve new problems. It is undoubtedly the most comprehensive and best standardized intelligence test available and as such should be considered the test of choice for assessing current intelligence level, provided the subject is able to tolerate the amount of testing involved.

The WAIS-R is not suitable for repeated measures over short time periods because of the practice effects involved. Ideally test/re-test intervals should be at least 6 months though shorter periods can be used if indicated clinically, particularly if the patient was considered previously to be poorly motivated and underachieving.

One of the limitations to the use of the WAIS-R is that only qualified psychologists are eligible to purchase it from the publishers. Correct administration and interpretation of the WAIS-R does require training and a good working knowledge of the principles involved, and since the test is such an invaluable tool clinically it is important to ensure that subjects are not inappropriately exposed to test items in a way that might invalidate future test results.

WAIS-R Short Forms
(Silverstein, 1982)

Silverstein (1982) reports a Two Subtest Short Form (Vocabulary and Block Design) and Four Subject Short Form (Vocabulary, Block Design, Arithmetic and

Picture Arrangement) of the WAIS-R, which have been derived from the original standardization data. Estimates of Full Scale IQ based on these subtest scores can be obtained from the tables provided in Silverstein's paper. As with the WAIS-R, these are grouped into different age ranges so that the IQs are age-corrected.

Utility

It is recommended that these short forms should not be used merely as a means of reducing testing time. Estimating IQs on the basis of fewer subtests will inevitably reduce the accuracy of the IQ estimate, and since the scatter of subtest scores tends to be higher in psychotic subjects than normals the chance of inaccuracy is correspondingly higher.

Despite the above limitations, the subtests of the short forms should be given first if the subject's co-operation is suspect; this will enable some interpretation of the results in terms of an overall IQ to be made even if the patient terminates the session prematurely.

Standard Progressive Matrices (SPM)
(Raven, 1938, latest manual 1988)

Standard Progressive Matrices is a test of deductive and inductive reasoning, and comprises 60 items in five sets of graded difficulty. Each item is a 3×3 matrix of shapes which change as they move across and down the grid according to some logical progression. The subject's task is to select from six or eight alternatives the shape that has been omitted from the bottom right-hand corner of the matrix. All items are attempted. The test is un-timed, but normally takes around 20 minutes. Although the test can be given in group form, an individual administration is preferable for psychotic patients as this enables the assessor to assess and evaluate concentration and motivation.

The raw scores are not converted into IQ equivalents but into percentile ranges, the ranges being defined by the 5th, 10th, 25th, 50th, 75th, 90th and 95th percentile points. These conversions are given for different age levels up to 65 years and so are corrected for age effects. However, the main table given in the manual for the adult population is based on data obtained during the 1940s and serious doubt must be raised about the validity of normative data of this age for today's population.

It would appear that the general level of intellectual functioning has been improving over the years so that tests standardized some time ago now overestimate levels of functioning relative to the normal population. For example, when the WAIS was re-administered as part of the WAIS-R standardization it was found that there had been an average increase of some 7.5 IQ points in the normal population over the previous 25 years, i.e. the average WAIS-IQ was now 107.5 In a recent study of low IQ chronic schizophrenic inpatients ($n = 46$) we found an average difference between RPM and WAIS-R results equivalent to approximately 15 IQ points, the RPM indicating higher levels of functioning. This is the more remarkable since there was evidence of significant intellectual deterioration in this group, and in these circumstances one would expect the WAIS-R to indicate higher IQ levels because of its greater dependence on previously acquired knowledge.

Reliability and validity
The SPM is a very well established and researched test with good reliability (generally 0.8 to 0.9) and validity as a measure of general intelligence (see manual for details). Furthermore, it appears to be largely free from the effects of cultural or educational factors.

Utility
The Matrices provide a measure of current, ongoing intellectual functioning that does not rely on previously acquired knowledge. It cannot be used to indicate level of functioning relative to the normal population (which is what an IQ figure represents) because reference to the standardization data may substantially over-estimate this level in today's population. However, it is a sensitive measure of general intelligence and as such is useful for measuring changes in levels of general intelligence over time. It is relatively quick and easy to administer and in view of this may be particularly useful for measuring change in patients with limited tolerance for testing or where a quicker test than the WAIS-R is indicated. Because of its speed and ease of administration the Matrices may also be the test of choice in a research programme where it is sufficient to establish that the groups are matched for current level of intelligence.

Coloured Progressive Matrices
(Raven, latest manual 1986)

This test is similar to the Standard Progressive Matrices but contains fewer and easier items. Standardization data (dating from the 1940s) is available for 65-85-year olds, with extrapolations for 90-100-year olds, and for sub-normal IQs across all age ranges.

Utility
The advantages and disadvantages of this test are similar to those of the Standard Progressive Matrices. Being short and with relatively simple items it is particularly suitable for frail elderly patients, or those of sub-normal intelligence.

Assessment of Intellectual Deterioration

Intellectual deterioration is not uncommon in psychotic subjects so an assessment of current level of intellectual functioning should not be considered complete without an estimate of premorbid level of functioning. When intelligence deteriorates the different aspects of intelligence do not deteriorate at the same rates, abilities based on previously acquired knowledge (notably verbal skills) are better maintained than abilities that depend on more ongoing, problem solving skills. This may be particularly relevant when drawing up a treatment or rehabilitation programme, for whilst good verbal skills may be advantageous socially, it is likely to be the ability to understand and cope with the problems that crop up in everyday life that will be the critical factor in determining success in a rehabilitation programme and/or living in the community.

In the absence of a formal cognitive assessment it is important to bear in mind the danger of overestimating the intellectual level and potential of a psychotic subject. Informal judgements about intelligence are based on intuitive evaluation of verbal skills; this is normally a good indicator for non-deteriorated subjects, but if a psychotic subject has deteriorated intellectually then his verbal skills will give a falsely high impression of his present capabilities. This, in turn, may lead to the setting of inappropriate goals and treatment programmes and to subsequent failure and frustration.

Studies comparing subjects on some particular aspect of cognitive functioning should be careful to match groups not only on a measure of present level of intelligence but also on premorbid level of intelligence. If the groups are not matched for extent of intellectual deterioration then any group differences that may occur in the target variables could be merely the manifestation of the differential decline of abilities that occurs in intellectual deterioration.

The need to match for extent of deterioration has implications for what constitutes an appropriate "control" group for studies involving psychotic subjects. Where there is evidence of intellectual deterioration in the psychotic subjects a "normal" control group may not be appropriate for studies of cognitive functioning.

The National Adult Reading Test (NART)
(Nelson, 1982; Nelson and Willison, 1991)

The NART provides an estimate of premorbid level of intelligence based on current reading level. Reading level correlates highly with IQ in normal subjects and is well maintained in the face of widespread intellectual decline. The NART comprises 50 words which are irregular in pronunciation so that they can only be read aloud correctly if the subject is, or has been, familiar with them. The total number of errors is recorded and from this score a WAIS or WAIS-R Full-Scale IQ equivalent is calculated. The test takes less than 5 min to administer.

Reliability and validity
High levels of inter-rater reliability (0.96-0.98) test-retest reliability (0.98) and split half reliability (0.93) have been reported. A number of studies have suggested that the NART provides a valid measure of premorbid IQ in cognitively impaired subjects, though it may underestimate premorbid IQ in more severely demented subjects or in those with a pronounced language deficit. (See Manual Supplement for review of statistical data).

The standard error of estimate associated with the estimated WAIS-R Full-Scale IQ equivalent is 8.6 points. The abnormality of the discrepancy between present IQ and estimated premorbid IQ (i.e. how often that size discrepancy or larger occurs in the normal population) is obtainable from actuarial tables presented in the Manual Supplement.

Utility

Reading is a relatively simple task and it is not obvious to the subject when he is making errors. The NART is quick to administer and well tolerated by patients, so it is recommended that it be used routinely when assessing intelligence.

If a patient is very thought disordered, so that his language is affected (e.g. producing neologisms), this may affect reading skills: in these circumstances the NART will tend to underestimate premorbid IQ level and hence underestimate the extent of intellectual deterioration. Similarly, if a patient is quite demented the NART may underestimate premorbid IQ level and hence underestimate the extent of intellectual deterioration.

Because of its speed and ease of administration the NART is often used as a measure of general intelligence in research projects when an approximate estimate of intelligence is sufficient. It is appropriate for this purpose providing there is no intellectual deterioration, but it is important to note that if there is intellectual deterioration then the measure provided will be of premorbid and not present level of functioning. For this reason the NART cannot be used to monitor intellectual changes over time.

Wechsler Adult Intelligence Scale – Revised
(Wechsler, 1981) (see page 89 for description)

In the absence of a measure of premorbid intellectual functioning, intellectual deterioration may be inferred from a discrepancy between the Verbal and Performance IQs of the WAIS-R in the direction of higher Verbal than Performance IQ. Items of the Verbal Scale rely more heavily on previously acquired knowledge than items of the Performance Scale and so the Verbal IQ declines more slowly than the Performance IQ. Within the Verbal Scale the Vocabulary and Information subtests will give the best indication of premorbid level of functioning, but even these are likely to be affected to some extent by the intellectual decline. Actuarial abnormality tables detailing the frequencies of occurrence of different V/P discrepancies in the normal population are given in Matarazzo and Herman (1985).

A right (non-dominant) hemisphere lesion will also tend to produce a Verbal/Performance IQ discrepancy in the direction of higher Verbal IQ, but in this case the Verbal IQ is retained at its premorbid level and there is not the characteristic scatter of subtest scores within the Verbal Scale. In psychotic patients a Verbal/Performance IQ discrepancy is much more likely to occur in the context of generalized intellectual deterioration than as a result of a unilateral, right hemisphere lesions.

Estimating Premorbid Intelligence from Academic and Occupational Histories and Demographic Variables
(Crawford et al.,1989)

Academic and occupational histories may provide some indication of intellectual level, particularly in the higher IQ ranges. As a rough rule of thumb an IQ of 120 plus would be needed for a traditional university degree, an IQ of 115 plus for GCE 'A' Levels.

If it is not possible to obtain an estimate of premorbid intelligence from test results or academic history, an estimate of WAIS IQ may be made on the basis of demographic variables according to the formula reported by Crawford *et al.* (1989):

Predicted WAIS FS IQ = 104.1 - 4.4 (social class) + 0.23 (age)
+ 1.4 (years of formal education) - 4.7 (sex) (S.e. est = 9.1)

Social class is determined using the OPCs Classification of Occupations (married females were classified by their husband's occupation), years of formal education includes 0.25 year for each year in day release or evening classes leading to formal qualification, and sex is a dummy variable coded with males = 1 and females = 2. An estimated WAIS-R equivalent of the predicted WAIS IQ may be obtained by deducting 7.5 points, though it should be noted that this conversion has an associated standard error of 7.8 points, which would effectively increase the standard error associated with the prediction.

Utility
This approach has the advantage of being suitable for patients who are unable/unwilling to undergo any formal testing. It may be particularly suitable for group studies, where inaccuracies in the individual case are of less concern than getting an overall view of the subjects, e.g. in group matching.

Dementia Rating Scale
(Mattis, 1973)

The Dementia Rating Scale was devised as a screening test to detect and discriminate between different levels of dementia and as such it is not sensitive to differences in levels of functioning in the normal, non-demented population. The test consists of a number of sub-sections to assess attention, perseveration (both verbal and motor), drawing ability, verbal and non-verbal abstraction, and verbal and non-verbal short-term memory. Normal elderly subjects find the questions easy and score at or near the ceiling of 144 points. It takes approximately 15 min to administer to normal, elderly subjects but may take up to 45 min with some demented patients.

Reliability and validity

Mattis reports a test/retest reliability over 1 week of 0.9 and clinical experience with Alzheimers Disease patients suggest a lawful decrement in score with duration of illness.

Utility

Because of the simplicity of the questions this scale may be useful for assessing psychotic subjects with very low levels of functioning for whom the standard tests of intelligence are too difficult. The test is well tolerated by patients and covers a comprehensive range of abilities.

The scale may be used clinically to assess dementia, especially by psychiatrists who do not have access to the WAIS-R, but more often it is used in research studies to match groups of subjects for dementia. It should be noted, however, that this is a test of present level of functioning rather than a measure of extent of dementia, i.e. it does not take into account differences in premorbid levels of functioning.

Assessment of Specific Cognitive Deficits

During an assessment of cognitive functioning certain features of a subject's responses, either quantitative or qualitative, may suggest a specific cognitive deficit, that is a deficit that occurs in the absence of any generalized loss or one that occurs in the presence of generalized loss but to a degree that is over and beyond that expected from the degree of generalized loss. The WAIS-R has potential for picking up specific deficits because it covers such a wide range of functions but it was constructed to be a test of general intelligence, not a neuropsychological screening test, and the subtests were selected because they provided good measures of general rather than specific factors of intelligence. Unless they are gross, specific cognitive deficits are usually apparent in the WAIS-R as qualitative rather than quantitative features of responses, and the assessor would need to have some experience with neuropsychological work to be able to detect them. If a specific deficit is suspected, then this may be investigated further using neuropsychological tests devised for this purpose (Lezak, 1983). (See also Chapter 12 of this book).

If cognitive impairment occurs in the psychoses it is usually a generalized impairment, affecting a wide range of functions. Nevertheless, some cognitive deficits may require an assessment that is independent of, or in addition to, the general assessment of intellectual status because of the potential impact of these deficits on treatment or lifestyle. Two such deficits are those of language comprehension and memory.

Assessment of Speed of Functioning

Cognitive speed is inversely related to negative symptomatology in chronic schizophrenia (Nelson *et al.*, 1990). Speed is an aspect of cognitive functioning that may be particularly sensitive to illness factors and drug effects and as such speed tests can be useful in monitoring progress over time.

Adult Memory and Information Processing Battery (AMIPB)
(Coughlan and Hollows, 1985)

The two information processing tests from this battery give measures of motor and cognitive speed cancellation task that takes less than 2 minutes to complete. The first test of cognitive speed comprises arrays of 5×2 digit numbers and the subject's task is to cross out the second highest number in each array. In the second test the subject compares strings of 4 and 5 digits and has the task of crossing out the additional digit appearing in the longer string. Each of these tests takes approximately 6 minutes to complete. There are good normative data from 180 subjects at different age levels, normative scores being given for the 2nd, 10th, 25th, 50th, 75th and 90th percentile levels. There are two parallel versions of the test.

Reliability and validity
Parallel form reliabilities range from 0.81 to 0.89 for these tests.

Language Comprehension

Subjects who have difficulty comprehending the spoken word are often assumed to be deaf, or their lack of responsiveness is attributed to their illness. But if there is extensive intellectual impairment the subject may have difficulty understanding even quite simple questions and statements, and in the case of very severe impairment, comprehension may be so affected that language has ceased to be an effective means of communication. Most assessments of symptomatology rely on the patient's responses to verbal questions, and treatment may depend on the patient following instructions and/or advice. Clearly it is very important in these situations to know how much a patient understands of what is said to him.

If the subject is suspected of being deaf, it is simple but effective to write down the question. Reading is well maintained in dementia and subjects will normally spontaneously read the questions aloud, even if they have lost the ability to comprehend what they read. Alternatively, if the subject is able to do a very simple verbal task, for example repeating two digits or pointing to common objects, then a crude test for deafness can be made by lowering the volume of the examiner's voice as the test is continued.

If comprehension is suspect, open ended questions should be used rather than questions requiring a "yes" or "no" answer. Although inappropriate answers may not necessarily be due to poor comprehension it is reasonable to assume from appropriate answers that the questions have been understood. If the patient does not reply to open ended questions it may be necessary to resort to yes/no questions, but in these circumstances the answers should not be taken at face value without attempting to check their validity. One way of doing this is to ask the questions in different ways such that appropriate "yes" and "no" answers are required for consistency.

In ordinary conversation or during a psychiatric interview, it may be difficult to determine whether a patient's poor or inappropriate responses are due to lack of comprehension *per se* or due to the effects of psychotic symptoms, such as poverty of thought, mutism, depression or thought disorder. In these circumstances a formal assessment of comprehension is recommended.

Modified De Renzi Token Test
(Coughlan and Warrington, 1978)

This is a modified and shortened version of the De Renzi and Vignolo (1962) Token Test: it takes less than 5 min to administer. The subject is given 15 commands using the coloured shapes of the Weigl Sorting Test, e.g. "Put the green square beside the red circle". Normative data are given for patients with left and right hemisphere lesions as well as 52 normal controls. Most normal subjects score 14 or 15 on this test, with 96% of subjects scoring 12 or more.

Reliability and validity
No reliability data are given. The test has good content validity.

Utility
The Modified Token Test is best used clinically as a semi-formal test for comprehension difficulties. Performance on this test may be adversely affected by poor short-term (immediate repetition) memory and distractability.

Simplified Token Test

If a patient is unable to respond to any of the questions of the Modified Token Test then the majority of the coloured shapes should be removed, leaving just the four different coloured squares. His response to very simple questions, such as "Give me the green one" or "Touch the blue one", will give some qualitative indication of the level of language comprehension that remains. The vast majority of psychotic patients will be able at least to identify the different colours, so failure to respond at this level may suggest lack of co-operation rather than comprehension loss.

Memory

Memory impairment is a common feature of intellectual impairment, indeed poor memory is often the first presenting feature of generalized cognitive loss. At a practical level, memory impairment in a psychotic patient may be particularly important because of its implications for his ability to follow a treatment programme or to cope with everyday living tasks.

Although specific memory deficits in neurological patients may respond well to remedial therapy (Wilson and Moffat, 1984) memory deficits occurring as part of a more widespread intellectual loss tend not to be so responsive because most therapies require the use of other cognitive skills to compensate for the memory loss. Even if those other cognitive skills are intact, learning to use them in a compensatory way requires effort and considerable motivation. Subjects whose memory loss occurs as part of a generalized intellectual impairment may be able to learn practical ways of avoiding reliance on memory, such as the use of a diary, but even this may well require a level of organization and motivation that is beyond the psychotic patient. If the psychotic patient is unable to compensate for his memory impairment it may be more profitable to consider how the environment might be modified so as to minimize the effects of the poor memory rather than trying to modify the patient's behaviour directly.

When evaluating a patient's memory it can be useful to obtain reports from relatives or staff about how his memory appears to be functioning in everyday life, as well as asking the patient for his own impression. Assessment of memory in the formal test situation does not always confirm the reports of memory functioning in everyday life. The formal assessment is relatively short and the presence of the examiner may ensure a level of concentration and motivation over the short time period that is not given to everyday tasks. In this case one would get a higher estimate of memory functioning from the formal test situation than one would from reports of everyday life. The occurrence of these discrepancies may have implications for deciding whether a memory loss has an organic or functional basis. Other factors that may influence this decision include the patients's behaviour in the test situation and any discrepancies that may occur between the different ways of assessing memory, for the example between recall and recognition measures.

Adult Memory and Information Processing Battery (AMIPB)
(Coughlan and Hollows, 1985) (see also page 97)

The Story Recall is similar to the passage in the Wechsler Memory Scale and consists of a short story broken into 28 ideas which are used for scoring. The story is read to the subject who recalls it in as much detail as he can, immediately after hearing it and then half an hour later. It takes less than 5 min to administer (plus the half hour test-retest interval). The Figure Recall is similar to the Rey Osterreith Figure and consists of a complex geometric figure which has first to be copied and then to be recalled immediately and then half an hour later. It takes 5 to 10 min to administer (in addition to the half hour test-retest interval), but scoring may be difficult and unreliable if the figure is badly distorted.

These are also list learning and figure learning subtests, but these require more sustained effort and as such may be unsuitable for poorly motivated subjects.

There are good normative data from 180 subjects at different age levels, normative scores being given for the 2nd, 10th, 25th, 50th, 75th and 90th percentile levels. There are two parallel versions of the tests.

Reliability and validity

Parallel form reliability for the Story and Figure Recall tests are in the region of 0.6 for immediate and delayed recall. This is a very conservative way of measuring test reliability and one would expect higher test-retest reliability if the same form were used: there are no data on practice effects using the same form. No inter-rater reliability figures are given in the manual, but experience in our department has suggested that although raters generally agree to within a couple of points for the story, scores may differ by 10 or more points for the figure, especially if it is badly distorted.

Utility

These tests of immediate and delayed recall are well standardized and the parallel forms enable re-testing to take place over a short interval.

However, the difficulty in scoring badly distorted figures suggest that this subtest may not be reliably scored in patients with poor visual memory.

The tests are quite short but they do require co-operation and some sustained effort on the part of the subject. Memory tested by recall generally demands more effort than memory tested by recognition or cueing techniques, and as such the AMIPB recall tests may be particularly susceptible to the effects of poor motivation and concentration, features often found in psychotic patients. Although recognition memory may give a better indicator of memory potential than recall memory, in practice much of the memory needed in everyday life is recall memory and so a measure of recall memory may reflect more accurately his actual level of memory in practical situations.

Recognition Memory Test
(Warrington, 1984)

The Recognition Memory Test is a forced choice recognition test of verbal (word) and visual (facial) memory which was devised to detect minor memory deficits in neuropsychological work. In the verbal memory subtest the subject is presented with 50 common, low imagery words which he judges for "pleasantness": this judgement forces the subject to attend to the word and to process it semantically. The Recognition Test follows immediately and consists of 50 word pairs, each being a word from the original list plus a distractor item. In the visual memory subtest a similar procedure is followed using 50 unfamiliar male faces. The whole test takes approximately 15 min to administer to normal subjects, but it may take considerably longer if subjects find it difficult to choose their responses.

The raw scores are converted into percentile ranges, the ranges being defined by the 5th, 10th, 25th, 50th, 75th, 90th and 95th percentile points. These conversions are given for three age ranges, less than 40, 40-55 and 55+ years. There is an abnormality table for word/faces discrepancy scores which describes how often discrepancies between the words and faces subtests occurred in the normal, standardization population.

Reliability and validity
The test was standardized on 310 adult subjects. No reliability data are given but the results from patients with unilateral brain lesions demonstrated the validity of the test for detecting memory deficits and for lateralizing lesions according to material specific deficits.

Utility
Testing memory by recognition techniques tends to be less affected by factors such as anxiety, depression or poor motivation than testing memory by recall, and in this respect the RMT may provide a better measure of memory potential than the AMIPB tests. Recognition tasks often appear to the subject to be easier and to require less effort than recall tasks but the length of the RMT may prove daunting to some psychotic subjects who may refuse to complete the long stimulus presentation stage. In this case the easier tests of the Rivermead Behavioural Memory Test (see below) may be used, but where subjects will complete testing the RMT is preferable in that it is sensitive to different levels of memory function across the whole normal range.

Rivermead Behavioural Memory Test (RBMT)
(Wilson et al., 1985)

This is a battery of 12 tests from which the Picture Recognition (approximately 3 min to administer) and Faces Recognition (approximately 2 min to administer) tests are particularly recommended. These tests were devised to detect and measure memory impairment and as such are not sensitive to differences in the normal memory range because of ceiling effects.

The Picture Recognition Test consists of 10 pictures of common objects which are presented to the subject for naming. After a few minutes these 10 pictures are presented again, mixed up with an equal number of new pictures, and the subject is asked whether he has seen each picture before. The Faces Recognition Test is conducted similarly with five faces, which the subject judges to be old or young. The score for each test is the number of items correctly recognized minus the number of false positives, (i.e. the number of new items incorrectly "recognized"). Only 1% of the normal population scores nine or less on the Picture Recognition Test: 9% of the normal population scores four or less on the Faces Recognition Test, with 2% of these scoring three or less.

The tests were standardized on 118 subjects: there are four parallel forms of the test.

Reliability and validity
Parallel form reliabilities for the whole RBMT were in the 0.8 to 0.9 range. The validity of the test in memory impaired subjects was established against the Recognition Memory Test (Warrington, 1984) and the Paired Associate Learning

Test (Inglis, 1957) and against rating of memory impairment from everyday life made by patients, their relatives and staff. Correlations between the RBMT and these variables were in the 0.4 to 0.7 range.

Utility

The RBMT was devised to provide a measure which would reflect severity of memory problems in everyday life rather than assess particular memory systems or localize cerebral lesions. The Picture Recognition and Faces Recognition Tests are short and easy and it requires only one or two errors to be made to indicate poor memory. Furthermore, with this type of recognition procedure, subjects are not aware of making errors and as such find the tests pleasant to do. These features make these tests ideal for use with psychotic patients who cannot complete the Recognition Memory Test, and although they cannot assess level of memory across the normal range they can screen for memory impairment which is severe enough to have implications for treatment programmes and everyday life. The four parallel forms of the test permit retesting over short periods.

Other Deficits

Research workers are increasingly turning to neuropsychological tests and techniques to provide information about specific cognitive deficits associated with the psychoses that may have implications for aetiology. The reader is recommended to consult Lezak (1983) for information about more specific neuropsychological tests that have been developed for their sensitivity to particular cognitive deficits and/or to the effects of circumscribed cerebral dysfunction. See Chapter 12 for information about discriminating between organic and affective psychoses, and the use of cognitive assessment in this difficult task.

References

Berg, E.A. (1948). A simple objective test for measuring flexibility in thinking. *Journal of General Psychology, 39*, 15-22

Bilder, R.M., Degreef, G., Pandurangi, A.K. *et al.* (1988). Neuropsychological deterioration and CT scan findings in chronic schizophrenia. *Schizophrenia Research, 1*, 37-45.

Canavan, A.G.M., Dunn, G. and Mcmillan, T.M. (1986). Principal components of the WAIS-R. *British Journal of Clinical Psychology, 25*, 81-85.

Coughlan, A.K. and Hollows, S.E. (1985). "The Adult Memory and Information Processing Battery (AMIPB)". Published by and obtainable from A.K. Coughlan, St James' University Hospital, Beckett Street, Leeds, LS9 7TF.

Coughlan, A.K. and Warrington, E.K. (1978). Word-comprehension and word-retrieval in patients with localized cerebral lesions. *Brain, 101*, 163-185.

Crawford, J.R., Stewart, L.E., Cochrone, R.H.B., Foulds, J.A., Besson, J.A.O. and Parker, D.M. (1989). Estimating premorbid IQ from demographic variables; regression equations derived from a UK sample. *British Journal of Clinical Psychology, 28*, 275-278.

DeRenzi, E. and Vignolo, L.A. (1962). The Token Test: a sensitive test to detect deceptive disturbances in aphasics. *Brain*, **85**, 665-678.

Goldstein, G. (1986). The neuropsychology of schizophrenia. *In* "Neuropsychological Assessment of Neuropsychiatric Disorders". (Eds I. Grant and K. Adams). Oxford University Press, Oxford.

Heaton, R.K. and Crowley, T.J. (1981). Effects of psychiatric disorders and the somatic treatments on neuropsychological test results. *In* "Handbook of Clinical Neuropsychology". (Eds S.B. Filskov and T.J. Boll), pp. 481-525. Wiley-Interscience, New York.

Inglis, J. (1957). An experimental study of learning and memory function in elderly patients. *Journal of Mental Science*, **103**, 798-803.

Johnstone, E.C., Owens, D.G.C., Gold, A. *et al.* (1981). Institutionalisation and the defects of schizophrenia. *British Journal of Psychiatry*, **139**, 195-203.

Lezak, M.D. (1983). "Neuropsychological Assessment". 2nd Edn. Oxford University Press, New York.

Matarazzo, J.D. (1972). "Wechsler's Measurement and Appraisal of Adult Intelligence". 5th Edn. Williams and Wilkins, Baltimore.

Matarazzo, J.D. and Herman, D.O. (1985). Clinical uses of the WAIS-R: Base rates of differences between VIQ and PIQ in the WAIS standardization sample. *In* "Handbook of Intelligence". (Ed. B. Wolman), pp. 899-932. John Wiley and Son, New York.

Mattis, S. (1976). Mental status examination for organic mental syndrome in the elderly patient. *In* "Geriatric Psychiatry". (Ed. L. Bellack and T.B. Karasu). Grune and Stratton, New York.

Nelson, H. E. (1982). "National Adult Reading Test (NART)". NFER-Nelson.

Nelson, H.E. and Willison, J. (1991). "National Adult Reading Test (NART)". 2nd Edn. NFER-Nelson.

Nelson, H.E., Pantelis, C., Carruthers, K., Speller, J., Baxendale, S. and Barnes, T.R.E. (1990). Cognitive functioning and symptomatology in chronic schizophrenia. *Psychological Medicine*. **20**, 357-365.

Payne, R.W. and Gwynne-Jones, H. (1957). Statistics for the investigation of individual cases. *Journal of Clinical Psychology*, **13**, 115-121.

Raven, J.C. (1958), "Standard Progressive Matrices". H.K. Lewis, London.

Raven, J.C. (1962). "Coloured Progressive Matrices". H.K. Lewis, London.

Reading Test Types, Keeler Ltd. 21-27 Marylebone Lane, London W1.

Shapiro, M.B. and Nelson, E.H. (1955). An investigation of the nature of cognitive impairment in co-operative patients. *British Journal of Medical Psychology*, **28**, 239-256.

Silverstein, A.B. (1982). Two- and four- subtest short forms of the Wechsler Adult Intelligence Scale – Revised. *Journal of Consulting and Clinical Psychology*, **50**, 415-418.

Warrington, E.K. (1984). "Recognition Memory Test". NFER-Nelson.

Wechsler, D. (1981). "Wechsler Adult Intelligence Scale" – Revised. The Psychological Corporation.

Wilson, B., Cockburn, J. and Baddeley, A. (1985). "The Rivermead Behavioural Memory Test". Thames Valley Test Company.

Wilson, B.A. and Moffat, N. (Eds.) (1984). "Clinical Management of Memory Problems". Croom Helm, London.

Zimmerman, I.L. and Woo-Sam, J.M. (1973). "Clinical Interpretation of the Wechsler Adult Intelligence Scale". Grune and Stratton, New York.

8. The Assessment of Subjective Experience and Insight

Brigid MacCarthy and Peter Liddle

It is traditionally accepted that there is a dissociation between the patient's subjective experience and observable behaviour in schizophrenia. In the case of core psychotic symptoms, this dissociation exists virtually by definition, since psychotic symptoms are taken to involve defective testing of reality. A "transformation of one's total awareness of reality" (Jaspars, 1913) is axiomatic to delusional experience. Thus in the International Pilot study of Schizophrenia, (WHO, 1973), the commonest recorded sign or symptom was lack of insight. In recent years descriptive psychiatry has tried to define static categories of phenomena to aid diagnosis and design methodical treatments (Strauss, 1989). Meanwhile biological formulations of aetiology have prompted schizophrenia research to refine its objective assessment techniques to aid the search for functional and anatomical abnormalities. This approach tends to emphasize a view of the patient as a passive victim of a process. As a result, there has been a tendency to undervalue patients' own descriptions of the illness, and to underestimate the degree of insight shown by many sufferers during its course. It is often assumed that their descriptions will be unreliable or invalid, and that lack of insight is absolute and unvarying during episodes of illness (Heinrichs et al., 1985).

However, the patient's own descriptions are potentially valuable, because the experiences to which they refer play an important part in determining how the illness is coped with. The quality of subjective experiences can influence the patient's willingness to take antipsychotic medication as well as form a basis for developing self-management strategies to minimize disability and vulnerability to external stress.

During the past decade, a growing number of studies of the subjective experiences of people with schizophrenia have demonstrated that such information can be reliable and valid. They have also provided insights into the nature of the disorder itself which suggest the need for a new "dynamic" approach to schizophrenia, which takes account of temporal and interactional processes.

Studies relying on retrospective accounts of patients in remission have shown that more than 60% of sufferers were able to recall the onset of episodes of acute disturbance. Patients could detail the order of emergence of prodromal symptoms, and were able to identify external stressors and coping strategies they had used to deal with particular symptoms (McCandless-Glimcher et al., 1986; Breier and Strauss, 1983). Donlon and Blacker (1973) and Doherty et al. (1978) argued that the onset of an episode of schizophrenia followed orderly and recognizable stages. Frankly psychotic symptoms, with their attendant diminution of insight emerged a week or more after the patient had experienced early signs such as anxiety, depression and agitation. These findings suggest that patients can and should be actively involved in the management of their illness, including seeking extra help on their own initiative, when early warning signs occur. A number of scales have been developed to systematize the monitoring of these early signs and will be discussed in detail below. As some of these studies have been conducted retrospectively, the reliability of patients' accounts must be open to doubt in the same way that all retrospective data are. However, findings from studies which include prospective samples indicate that although awareness of the unrealistic nature of some beliefs and experiences dwindles in the final prodromal stages (e.g. Birchwood *et al.*, 1989), and acutely ill patients have difficulty making sense of questions about the quality of their experiences, remitted patients' accounts are stable over time and are consistent with external observations (Cutting and Dunne, 1989).

Studies which have paid careful attention to the fixity of delusional beliefs have challenged the assumption that lack of awareness of psychotic phenomena is axiomatic or universal. When conviction is treated as a dimensional rather than all or nothing attribute, fluctuations over time (Garety, 1985; Brett-Jones *et al.*, 1987) have been reported. Donlon and Blacker (1973) also found some indication that insight can return, and recovery proceed through the same sequence of stages as onset, but with the sequence running in reverse.

Traditionally, clinicians interview patients most closely during the extreme acute phase of their illness, when they are least likely to be capable of discussing their experiences coherently or of showing insight into the idiosyncratic quality of their beliefs. Few clinicians have the opportunity or perhaps see the purpose of developing the long-term trusting relationships which informed the clinical richness of the observations of Bleuler (1911) or Arieti (1974). Although the lack of insight which is assumed to define psychotic experience, may characterize most patients some of the time, and a few patients all of the time, evidence shows such marked variability both within and between patients suffering from schizophrenia (Liddle, 1986; Strauss, 1989) as to make that assumption quite unjustified.

Definitions of "Insight"

A bewildering array of phenomena have been investigated under the rubric of "awareness"'or "insight", which has often led to contradictory findings. In the context of psychotic illnesses, "insight" has traditionally been equated with evidence that the patient shares the clinician's perception of reality: lack of insight therefore amounts to maintaining an idiosyncratic perception of reality with a degree of conviction which is not open to disconfirming evidence (Garety, 1985). However, there are two relatively independent ways of defining lack of insight, and a third, meta-level evaluation of experience, each of which has been cited by different authors as the core experience of insight.

First, a patient may be capable of reporting private experiences accurately, but fail to evaluate the experiences in ways which achieve consensus with others, particularly the treating clinician. When insight is thus defined, it has provoked criticisms for being open to ideologically motivated abuse. An absolute line cannot be drawn between culturally normative and abnormal states of mind or beliefs, although genuinely controversial cases are rare. Many delusional beliefs lie on a boundary between concretely expressed metaphors conveying emotional truths, and full-blown delusional ideas with no meaningful content (Arieti, 1974). Since these experiences have no observable correlate, it is difficult to establish the validity of assessment of insight defined in this way.

Secondly, a patient may be unable to monitor or make accurate reports of subjective experiences but, were they able to, they would share the consensus view of the abnormality of the experiences. Lack of insight of this kind is more likely to occur in respect of deficit states, observable behavioural changes and external "events" or stressors.

The third, meta-level definition of insight refers to the patient's understanding or acceptance of a psychological explanation or illness model to account for their experiences and endorsement of professionals' views about need for treatment. However, to consider the full extent of the subjective experience and insight of people suffering from schizophrenia, assessments of phenomena beyond the core signs and symptoms of the disorder are needed. In turn the information gathered during such wider assessments is needed to support the design of self-management treatment programmes (see Scales reviewed below).

Barriers to insight specific to schizophrenia

Aetiological theories suggest reasons why people suffering from schizophrenia should be particularly likely to lack insight. Early psychoanalytic theories proposed that positive symptoms were formed to express or resolve intolerable conflicts. Since they are defences it is argued that the sufferer will resist recognizing the irrationality of their content. A modification of this argument, developed by Mayer-Gross and others since (McGlashan, 1987) is that a process of sealing-over may take place, when recovering patients try to forget psychotic experiences or relegate them to a separate and enclosed part of their past.

Experimental psychology provides explanations for deficits in the first and second types of insight. Self-evaluation and self-monitoring respectively (Breier and Strauss, 1983) may be peculiarly limited by the schizophrenic process itself. Frith and Done (1988; 1989) suggest that core impairments in schizophrenia may reflect inaccurate monitoring of behaviour and failure to discriminate intentional from unintentional acts. These failures may be associated with omissions in very short-term memory (Frith and Done, 1989). Both posited mechanisms would be likely to impair self-monitoring and evaluation.

Methodological issues

It is difficult to establish the reliability or validity of patients' own reports, particularly if the phenomena are purely private. Comparisons have been made with clinicians' observations, which is to assume that the clinicians' judgements are necessarily veridical. However, the validity of clinicians' judgements is open to question for a number of reasons. The information gathered in a clinical interview, where often the patient and clinician are relative strangers, is likely to be partial (Brewin *et al.,* 1990) and the quality of information obtained, especially about such delicate issues, will be strongly related to the intimacy and trust established. Also, behaviours assumed to be associated with the primary or core symptoms of the disease process may sometimes be comparatively adaptive attempts to cope with other more central impairments (e.g. Hemsley, 1977).

There are three main strategies capable of assessing subjective experience: global standardized scales, semi-structured interviews, and process measures. They generate progressively more specific data. However, even the least generalized measures can be used sufficiently systematically to provide group as well as individual data (Morley, 1989). At each level of specificity, a range of methods have been used, requiring more or less direct self-report from the patient: at one extreme, questionnaires or forms are completed independently by the patient and at the other extreme, assessments have been based on purely external observation, without any direct participation from the patient.

The majority of the instruments reviewed below are structured, global scales, containing a fixed number of questions with a completely pre-determined format. These scales clearly produce the greatest amount of generalizable information, but because of the unique quality of the subject matter, may fail to capture significant variation. At a greater level of specificity, a number of instruments provide moderately standardized procedures for making individualized, targetted assessments: here semi-structured interviews, personalized questionnaires and content analyses using pre-determined categories have been used. Finally, process measures, establishing individualized baselines and recording variation over time in targetted phenomenon have also been used.

The Assessment Procedures

Subjective Awareness of Abnormal Mental Processes

In many cases of schizophrenia, overt psychotic episodes are superimposed upon relatively stable periods in which the patient suffers a degree of residual impairment. This suggests that schizophrenia is characterized by persistent perhaps subtle, abnormalities in mental processing which predispose the patient to become psychotic when subjected to stress. Bleuler (1911) considered that underlying persistent abnormalities were reflected in observable abnormalities which he called fundamental symptoms. These include disorders such as looseness of associations and flattened affect. Bleuler claimed that these fundamental symptoms are present in all cases and at all phases of the illness, although in many cases they are not easy to detect at any stage of the illness.

Nonetheless, several strands of evidence suggest that a large proportion of schizophrenic patients do have subjective awareness of subtle abnormalities of mental processing in both acute and chronic phases of the illness. These phenomena occur in individuals at risk for schizophrenia, are especially prevalent during the prodromal phases of a psychotic episode, and are common during stable phases of the illness. Scales have been designed to measure the subjective experience of these abnormalities at each phase.

(i) Scales for Pre-psychotic Phenomena

The following scales were developed to detect putative pre-psychotic phenomena in individuals who are possibly at risk of suffering from schizophrenia.

Social-Anhedonia Scale
(Chapman and Chapman, 1987)

This scale measures the sustained deficit in the enjoyment of social interactions, which might be a precursor of the negative symptoms of schizophrenia.

The Perceptual Aberration – Magical Ideation Scale
(Chapman and Chapman, 1987) (see also Chapter 3)

This scale includes items such as illusions, hypnogogic hallucinations and aberrant beliefs which might be precursors of positive schizophrenic symptoms.

Utility
The power of these symptoms assessed in the above two scales to predict subsequent schizophrenia is not clearly established.

(ii) Scales for Prodromal Symptoms

Several investigators have developed scales for measuring symptoms experienced in the prodromal phase of a psychotic episode. The possibility that these symptoms can be accurately assessed has been exploited in the development of innovative treatment strategies where the patient has to play a responsible role in monitoring and identifying early signs, before insight is lost (Herz and Melville, 1980; Hirsch and Jolley, 1989)

Early Signs Questionnaire
(Herz and Melville, 1980)

This is a 32 item scale covering feeling, thinking and perception. The questionnaire is administered in a standardized manner and the severity of each item is scored on a five point scale.

Validity
Seventy per cent of patients were found to be aware of prodromal symptoms in the days or weeks preceding overt psychotic relapse.

Utility
Some of the items, such as lability of mood, altered energy level and impaired concentration are not specific to schizophrenia, while others assess attentuated forms of overt schizophrenic phnenomena.

Early Signs Scale (ESS)
(Birchwood et al., 1989)

The Early Signs Scale (ESS) was developed to monitor changes in key symptoms in the 2 weeks preceding a putative relapse. Forms are completed retrospectively at 2 week intervals, but they anticipate that monitoring will be continuous. Thus significant exacerbations are not masked by the presence of persistent symptoms, since each individual has a clearly established base-line. To compensate for declining insight in the prodromal phase, the scale is completed in a phenomenological version by the patient, and in a behavioural version by a close relative. It comprises 34 items, rated on four-point scales, running from "not a problem/zero times in a week", to "marked problem/at least once a day". These items cluster in four sub-scales with high proven internal consistency: "anxiety/agitation" (e.g. irritable; sleep problems), "depression/withdrawal" (e.g. quiet, poor appetite) "disinhibition" (e.g. restless, stubborn) and "incipient psychosis" (e.g. odd behaviour; says is being watched).

Reliability and validity
The scales were subjected to rigorous psychometric scrutiny. Test-retest reliability achieved high correlations in both versions: $r = 0.98$ for the self-report version, and $r = 0.84$ for informants. Concurrent validity, established by asking subjects to complete a standardized self-report measure of psychopathology, was also high ($r > 0.74$ for all subscales). The scale achieved 79% overall accuracy in predicting relapse, with no false positives. This considerably improved on the ability of a standardized clinical interview administered with the same frequency to identify individuals in danger of relapse.

Utility
The authors suggest that the ESS is able to detect changes in non-psychotic phenomena which would not or could not be monitored by clinicians in routine follow-ups, but which are nevertheless useful markers of impending relapse.

(iii) Scales for Persisting Deficits

Huber and colleagues have described a subjectively experienced defect state which occurs in some schizophrenic patients, which they claim is more closely related to the neurological substrate of schizophrenia. In particular, they found evidence that the severity of the symptoms of this defect state, which they term the "basic disorder", is correlated with degree of enlargement of the cerebral ventricles.

Bonn Scale for the Assessment of Basic Symptoms (BSABS)
(Gross, 1985)

This scale consists of 106 items arranged in six categories: "dynamic deficiencies – direct minus symptoms", reflecting decreased capacity for physical and psychological activity; dynamic impressionability; "cognitive thought disorders", such as interference of thought, disturbed concentration and retardation of thought processes; "coenesthesias" (disturbed bodily sensations); "vegetative and motor disorders"; and "coping mechanisms". Defining criteria for each symptom are provided and a glossary provides comments. However, the interview is non-directive, without standardized questions, and item severity is not quantified.

Sub-Clinical Symptoms (Sub-S)
(Petho and Bitter, 1985)

The Sub-Clinical Symptoms scale was developed to assess the symptoms that occur in the residual phase of the illness. This scale contains a separate sub-scale for subjective experiences (comprising 19 items covering experiences such as nervousness, irritability, indecisiveness, reduced will power and sensitivity to weather) and a sub-scale for behavioural characteristics which includes nine observable abnormalities of behaviour such as disorders of appearance, irresponsibility and indifference.

Reliability and validity
They obtained good reliability for virtually all items of both scales. Using the Coefficient of Intercategory Reliability defined by Bartko and Carpenter (1976) as a measure of inter-rater reliability, Petho and Bitter (1985) obtained coefficients in the range 0.51 to 0.98 for the coefficient of reliability between pairs of raters, for all items of the scale except for two behavioural items: irresponsible (0.15) and unstable behaviour (0.28). Factor analysis indicated that the two scales measure clearly distinct aspects of the phenomena of psychosis.

Subjective Experience of Deficits in Schizophrenia (SEDS)
(Liddle and Barnes, 1988) (see also Chapter 5)

This scale includes the principal types of subjective abnormalities of mental processing reported by schizophrenic patients during relatively stable phases of the illness. It comprises 21 items arranged in five groups, namely abnormal thinking and concentration; disturbance of affect; impaired will and decreased energy;

disturbances of perception, coenesthesia and motor function and intolerance of stress. The assessment is based on a semi-standardized interview, with specified probe questions. For each item, the occurrence of the experience, the perceived disruption of activities, and the degree of distress are recorded, and overall severity of the symptom is scored on a five point scale ranging from "absent" to "severe". The items are defined in a glossary.

Reliability and validity

Liddle and Barnes demonstrated that the scale items are prevalent among chronic schizophrenic patients and can be scored with satisfactory reliability. They obtained values of Cohen's Kappa lying in the range 0.53 to 0.94 for all items of the scale.

Psychotic Phenomena

Here interest has focussed on patients' evaluation of phenomena, assessing their insight into the abnormal quality of their experiences or beliefs, rather than the accuracy of their awareness. None of the scales reviewed are structured or global, reflecting the need, dictated by the idiosyncratic nature of the material under observation, to tailor the assessment to individuals' particular ideas. This need has led to the development of some innovative techniques. Structured observation of patients' varying attitudes to their beliefs and experiences may provide both clinical and research tools, help to redefine diagnostic categories and indicate potential intervention strategies.

Subjective Experience of Schizophrenia
(Cutting and Dunne, 1989)

This is a "structured interview", developed to assess the recall of abnormalities in the process of psychological functioning during acute episodes of schizophrenia, such as disturbances to perception, attention and memory. No attempt is made to assess the contents of delusions or hallucinations and no attempt is made to assess current experience, because the authors found that acutely ill patients were unable to participate in the interview.

The interview contains seven relatively open-ended questions with accompanying probes concerning visual and auditory perception, language, attention, movement, thinking and space. No details of the scoring procedure are given.

Reliability and validity

In a validation study, patients whose schizophrenic symptoms had remitted at least one year previously were questioned about the first episode of their disorder and their responses compared with those of a matched group of depressed patients.

Only six out of 30 items scored discriminated significantly between the schizophrenic and depressed patients and one of these occurred more frequently among the depressed sample.

The authors rightly point out that the validity of such retrospective evidence is suspect. Case notes were scanned but could not provide validating evidence as changes in psychological processes had not been recorded.

Utility
In view of the difficulty of conducting the interview with patients currently suffering from schizophrenia, the unusual focus of the questions, the unproven validity of the retrospective data, and its inability to discriminate between psychotic and non-psychotic subjects, this exploratory instrument clearly needs further development before it will be of general use.

Personal Questionnaire Technique
(Brett-Jones et al., 1987) (see also Chapter 3)

The Personal Questionnaire technique (Shapiro, 1961) allows the measurement of change in symptoms specific to individual patients by scaling different levels of symptom intensity. Building on earlier work by Garety (1985) Brett-Jones (1987) used this technique to measure fluctuations in patients' anxieties and pre-occupation with their delusional beliefs. This approach emphasizes the dimensional nature of delusional beliefs, countering Jaspers' (1913) insistence that delusions are necessarily held with extraordinary conviction.

Conviction and pre-occupation are measured with a six-point ordinal scale, running from "I doubt that ..." to "I am absolutely certain that ..." for assessing conviction, and "I think about these things not at all ..." to "I think about these things absolutely all the time ..." for assessing pre-occupation. These anchors are defined by the researcher, but the specific content of the delusional belief is supplied by each patient. In the Brett-Jones *et al.* study, each patient was interviewed weekly until discharge or for a maximum of 6 months.

Reliability and validity
Inter-rater and test-retest reliability checks achieved weighted Kappa coefficients ranging from 0.75 to 0.89 (all $p < 0.002$), and in eight out of the nine cases, subjects' final ratings of conviction agreed with psychiatrists' assessments of delusional status.

Subjective Awareness of Observable Abnormalities and Deficits

Scale for the Assessment of Negative Symptoms (SANS)
(Andreasen, 1982) (see also Chapter 5)

A subjective item is included in each of the five sub-scales, which measure flatness of affect; poverty of speech; avolition/apathy; anhedonia/asociality; and attentional impairment. The subjective items assess the patient's awareness of each of these deficits.

Reliability and validity

The inter-rater reliability for the subjective items of SANS was satisfactory. Values of intraclass reliability were in the range 0.72 to 0.92. In her initial evaluation of the scale, Andreason (1982) reported that correlations between each of the subjective items and the relevant sub-scale score were low (0.25-0.6).

Utility

Because some correlations between subjective and objective measures were relatively low, Andreason omitted the subjective items from more recent versions of SANS. However, when Liddle (1986) administered SANS to a group of chronic schizophrenic patients in a stable phase of their illness, he obtained correlations in the same range as those of Andreason but found that some patients with observable flatness of affect were strongly aware of the phenomenon, and extremely distressed by it, while others were entirely unaware of the problem. The modest correlations at group level between subjectively and externally assessed phenomena, may mask a substantial relationship in a sub-group of cases. A single-case study reported by Bouricius (1989) using the same instrument, showed that clinicians also vary considerably in how closely their external ratings mirror those made by the patient. It may therefore be premature to abandon the subjective item from the SANS, when at least some of the information it yields may help to direct treatment efforts. In addition, careful assessment of patients' subjective awareness may delineate the underlying psychopathological processes which contribute to the observable phenomena assessed by SANS. In particular, observable items on which the assessment of avolition/apathy is based are mainly items concerned with persistence at work and other activities. The conclusion that poor performance is due to avolition depends on a judgement about unobservable aspects of mental functioning. Since the time of Kraeplin and Bleuler, impairment of volition has been considered an important feature of schizophrenia, and the lack of adequate means of measuring avolition is perhaps one of the major shortcomings of current techniques for measuring the psychopathology of schizophrenia.

Task Motivation and Problem Appraisal
(MacCarthy et al., 1986)

This instrument is based on Bandura's model of motivation "expectancy theory" (Bandura, 1977), and is designed to measure patients' appraisal of their functional difficulties and motivation to change their behaviour.

For each of 10 everyday and domestic tasks, patients are interviewed about whether they have a problem in performing the task, and how important, difficult and successful they thought their own efforts to complete the task would be. Answers are scored on 4-point scales, in which each point is clearly defined and printed on cards presented to the patient. Patients select their preferred answer by choosing one of the four cards.

Reliability and validity
In the MacCarthy *et al.* study, day-care staff accounts of patients' difficulties, using the same checklist, achieved 87% overall agreement with the patients.

Utility
The exercise demonstrated that patients were able to make internally consistent replies to questions assessing motivation and that they discriminated between lack of motivation and pragmatic reasons for their functional deficits.

Coping

The patient's conscious understanding of automatic or preferred coping responses is the important final stage of an active response to the disorder and is of immediate interest to clinicians seeking to work collaboratively with the patient. Patients' own accounts of their coping efforts have shown that clinicians need to discriminate carefully between basic defect states and behaviour which resembles outward signs of such states. This behaviour may represent coping efforts aimed at controlling other, more disabling symptoms (Falloon and Talbot, 1981; Hemsley, 1977; Thurm and Haefner, 1987). Results of systematic research can enhance clinicians' ability to advise patients about successful ways of coping, identify relationships between types of coping and possible underlying causal mechanisms or differentiate groups likely to respond most effectively to different treatment regimes (Breier and Strauss, 1983).

Coping Mechanisms for Persistent Auditory Hallucinations
(Falloon and Talbot, 1981)

This technique uses an unstructured interview to elicit accounts of behaviour, thoughts and feelings contingent on interference from auditory hallucinations. Examples of open-ended probes are given in the paper. Responses are classified as "behaviour change" (e.g. postural change, interpersonal contact, drug taking), manipulating "physiological arousal" (e.g. sleeping, stimulating music) or "cognitive strategies" (e.g. reduce attention to voices, accept voices). In the original study, adaptation to hallucinations was rated by a clinician, and correlated with the frequency with which types of coping was used. The best outcome was associated with using a limited number of strategies consistently, particularly when the patient was aware of environmental precipitants.

Utility
The strength of this study is the guidance given about the interview procedure and its specific focus on efforts to cope with a single phenomenon. However, no reliability data were reported for the system of classification. Examples quoted suggest that the allocation of specific strategies to categories was idiosyncratic and would be difficult to replicate.

Personal Coping Styles
(Cohen and Berk, 1985)

This is an open-ended interview, based on Herz and Melville's (1980) Early Signs Questionnaire in which coping strategies for specific problems are elicited. In the original study a vast number of strategies were identified, which were divided into nine categories: fighting back, time out, isolated diversion, social diversion, prayer, medical, use of drugs or alcohol, does nothing but feels helpless, does nothing but accepts symptoms. Examples are given of typical strategies within each category. These examples give the classification high face validity, but no further psychometric data are reported. Because the interview procedure has linked individual problems to specific strategies, the authors were able to show that there were systematic differences in preferred coping strategies between problems.

Self Control in Psychotic Disorders
(Breier and Strauss, 1983)

These authors argued that patients' self control efforts in the face of psychotic disorders can be analyzed in three phases: self-monitoring, self-evaluation and self-management. In what was effectively a series of single case studies, they found that a group of acutely ill patients could describe the process of monitoring and evaluating abnormal aspects of their experience, and that a majority could give an account of subsequent coping efforts. Self-management strategies included self-instruction, and increasing and decreasing behaviour. They hypothesized that differences in preferred coping strategies might be related to different pathology in information processing. The explicit application of a model to the processes they have investigated, and the attempt to link their findings to other explanatory models is an advantage of the study.

Utility
The procedure as it stands is only a systematizing of careful clinical observation. However, it could readily be developed into a more structured instrument allowing the collection of quantifiable information.

Coping Behaviour Questionnaire
(Boker et al., 1989)

A semi-structured interview was used to elicit strategies with reference to four areas of disturbance assessed and defined by a standardized questionnaire as routinized skills, perception, depression/anhedonia, and stimulus overload. Coping responses are divided into two main groups; harmless problem-solving-oriented behaviour, which includes "compensatory efforts aimed consciously and directly at eliminating the source of interference", and non-problem-solving-oriented behaviour, which included "all conscious attempts at avoidance, shielding and social withdrawal".

Reliability and validity
In the original study inter-rater agreement achieved 90% for this two-way classification. A more detailed classification into seven groups: "balancing out", "reinterpretation", "restructuring", "structuring", "shift in behaviour", "reality testing", and "behavioural stereotypes" is suggested, but no examples or psychometric data are given.

Utility
The strength of the original study lies in the structure imposed on the process of eliciting the coping data by using a standard questionnaire. The questionnaire itself is based on a coherent explanatory model and has an explicitly limited focus. The study also included a limited assessment of the reliability of the coping categories.

Coping in Schizophrenia
(Thurm and Haefner, 1987)

These authors conducted semi-structured interviews with 37 patients with a long history of schizophrenia, to establish their perceptions of vulnerability, risk of relapse and coping skills. Having established the patients' ability to identify stressors and prodromal symptoms, descriptions of coping strategies were elicited and coded, using content analysis, into categories reflecting their form and function. The coding system for strategies used to avoid relapse in the face of specific stressors had three categories: protecting the self from over-stimulation, getting involved in everyday life to balance over- and under- stimulation, and intrapsychic strategies. Strategies used to cope with emerging symptoms were coded into four categories: seeking help, intrapsychic methods, taking extra medication and "behavioural change".

Reliability and validity
Examples are cited for the first system, which suggests it has face validity, but no reliability data were reported for either system.

Utility
This study shares with the others reviewed in this section, the merit of linking elicited strategies to specific phenomena, but otherwise offers only limited details about procedure and materials.

Utility of scales uses to assess coping skills
The scales reviewed here have used, at best, semi-structured interviews to elicit information on coping. Some studies restrict the investigation to efforts to cope with core psychotic phenomena, others include prodromal symptoms or environmental stress. Patients' responses have then been categorized, using a *priori* systems or content-analysis. A general methodological weakness in this area is the lack of evidence on the reliability or validity of rating systems, making replication difficult.

External Stress

The vulnerability model of schizophrenia (e.g. Zubin *et al.*, 1985) argues that even minor variation in endogenous and exogenous factors, operating on an already vulnerable organism will predict when an individual will move in and out of acutely ill phases of a psychotic disorder. Psycho-social interventions have placed much emphasis on this model. Increasingly, these interventions require the active participation of the patient which in turn requires the patient to develop skills in accurately monitoring the external environment. Of interest particularly, is the patient's ability to assess the emotional atmosphere of the family and the occurrence of stressful events, since it has been shown that both factors play a vital role in predicting relapse (Thurm and Haefner, 1987).

(i) Family atmosphere

Very little research has looked at patients' perceptions of family atmosphere, and no studies of schizophrenic subjects have directly examined their awareness of the factors measured by the "Expressed Emotion" index, despite the enormous volume of work in recent years relating to this construct. The two published scales reviewed below have shown that it is a feasible and valid exercise to elicit patients' perceptions of family attitudes and outcome. The strong relationships found between their perceptions and outcome suggest that patients are aware of pathogenic influences in their home environment.

Family Interpersonal Perception Test
(Scott and Alwyn, 1978)

This test assesses the "tenability" of the patient's relationship with his parents. Patients and their parents complete adjective checklists, judging themselves, each other and the other's view of themselves on personality attributes such as "responsible", "confused" and "timid". Scores are calculated to reflect the ratio of "wellness" to "illness" and "nervousness" comparing different viewpoints.

Reliability and validity
In the original study it was found that when patients perceived negative features in their parents which their parents did not expect, they were likely to have left home during the two-and-a-half years follow-up period. Apart from this measure of predictive validity no other reliability or validity tests were reported.

Utility
The authors point out that the test and its scoring system does not assess accuracy of perception, but the extent to which patients and parents share a viewpoint. The complexity of the scoring system makes it difficult to sense what aspects of family functioning might be reflected by the measure until concurrent validity has been established.

The Parental Bonding Instrument (PBI)
(Parker et al., 1979)

This is a 25 item self-report questionnaire which asks subjects to rate their parents' attitudes and behaviour towards them in their first 16 years. Each item is rated on a 4-point scale, running from "very like" to "very unlike". Two subscale scores can be compiled to reflect the semi-independent dimensions of care and affection (e.g. "appeared to understand my problems and worries") and overprotection/control (e.g. "tried to make me dependent on him/her") that had been identified by factor analysis.

Reliability and validity
Test-retest reliability was assessed over a 3 week period, and split-half and inter-rater reliability was also assessed, for the two subscales separately. Correlation coefficients ranged between 0.63 and 0.88, and were all significant at the 0.001 level. Correlations between self-report scores and estimates of the same constructs made by clinicians following an interview were calculated. The correlation coefficient for the care measure was 0.77, while the correlation for overprotection was 0.48 for one rater, and 0.51 for a second rater. Patients' siblings completed the test at the same time, pretending to be the patients. The mean correlation coefficient was 0.46, suggesting that the scale is likely to reflect patients' perceptions more accurately than actual parent characteristics.

Utility
Some population norms are available. PBI ratings were found to be associated with the course of schizophrenia in the year following test administration (Warner and Atkinson, 1988). No further validation of the accuracy of recall of subjects has been attempted, so it is not clear whether the measure really reflects past or current interactions between patients and their parents.

(ii) Life-events

Research on the effect of life-events on the course of schizophrenia has, in contrast to the work on family atmosphere, been based mainly on subjects' own accounts. Since these studies have shown that high levels of stress are related to increased risk of relapse (Bebbington and Kuipers, 1988) this indirectly suggests that patients are able to monitor external life-event stress accurately. However, the veracity of reports made by people suffering from schizophrenia has not been tested directly, as it has in other disorders. As no scales have been designed specifically to assess major life-event stress in psychotic populations, none is reviewed in detail here.

Experiences of Precipitating Factors
(Thurm and Haefner, 1987)

The procedure used to elicit information and the subjects were the same as were used to establish their coping schema. Eighty-one per cent of their sample were able to identify at least one major risk factor. Three main types of stressor were identified: social-emotional (interpersonal conflicts and intense emotions in close relationships), social-cognitive (experiences leading to information overload and overstimulation), and absence of social stimulation. Positive changes were as likely to precipitate relapse as negative changes.

Reliability and validity
No reliability or validity data are reported.

Experience Sampling Method (ESM)
(de Vries and Delespaul, 1989; Csikszentmihalyi and Larson, 1987)

This innovative study used a self-report time sampling technique to gather information about the effect of social context on subjective experience. Very detailed information was obtained about the consequences, for nine psychotic individuals, of minor external daily stress. Patients carry electronic beepers which signal them, at 10 randomized times during the day, to complete report forms. These forms contained 19 7-point Likert scales, scored from "not at all" to "totally true". The items form four subsets with proven internal consistency: thinking (e.g. pleasant, clear), mood (e.g. cheerful, calm), physical concerns (e.g. hungry, tired) and schizophrenic symptoms (e.g. "I hear voices", "I can't get rid of my thoughts"). A further four open-ended questions establish where the patient was, what they were doing, who they were with and the contents of their thoughts.

Reliability and validity
Data were recorded for 80% of the sampling periods, and correlated $r > 0.70$ with information collected in a number of different ways, such as by retrospective diary-keeping, completion of standardized personality inventories and use of physiological measures.

Utility
Although completing the self-report forms was arduous, there were few missing data points. However, the coding of the open ended questions was reported to be time consuming and required lengthy subsequent discussions between researchers and patients. The scale provides rich information about the timing and stimuli which precede psychotic phenomena and about patients' coping responses. Although the procedure does allow for analysis of group data, the authors anticipate that time series analyses will provide clinically useful information on a case by case basis.

Insight into the Nature of the Illness

Attempts to measure the perspective the patient has on the experience of illness as a whole, has been most reasonably summarized as, the patient's awareness that he or she is suffering from a mental illness (Heinrichs *et al.*, 1985). In practice, assessments have operationalized this idea in rather curious ways.

Roback and Abramowitz (1979) asked psychotic subjects to choose between alternative explanations for a set of inter-personal scenarios. A high "insight" score was obtained by selecting a high-consensus explanation which attributed events to psychological characteristics of the actors.

Heinrichs *et al.* (1985) conducted a study in which the assessment of early insight during episodes of decompensation was based entirely on judgements made by personnel reviewing progress notes. Validity for these ratings was established by interviewing clinicians retrospectively for a sub-sample of cases in the study, achieving concordance in 90% of cases. Thus, although the operational definition of insight used in this study, which was quoted above, was conceptually reasonable, clarification of the validity of the assessments is needed.

Insight and Treatment Attitude Questionnaire
(McEvoy et al., 1989)

This is an 11 item questionnaire that assesses the patient's insight in terms of the congruence of his judgements about his experiences and need for treatment with the judgement of involved health professionals. The questionnaire is administered as an interview and verbatim responses are rated for good/partial/no insight.

Reliability and validity
In the original study inter-rater reliability was high ($r = 0.82, p < .001$). Construct validity, checked by correlating scores with an open interview and medication compliance, was also high ($r = 0.85, p < .001$).

The Schizophrenia Experience
(Soskis and Bowers, 1969)

Subjects are asked to indicate whether they agree with each of 10 statements about the usefulness of understanding the illness compared to forgetting about it.

Reliability and validity
No reliability or validity data were reported in the original study, but believing in the positive value of insight was found to relate to long-term adjustment.

Conclusion

Investigators have approached the assessment of subjective experiences of patients with schizophrenia from a variety of perspectives, which is reflected in the multiplicity of scales that have been developed. While there is clear evidence that these patients' subjective experiences can be assessed reliably, the utility of many of the scales has not been established. Hence, unsurprisingly, few of the scales have been widely used.

The diversity of subjective experiences in schizophrenia diminishes the relevance of a strict insistence on standardized assessments. Nonetheless, for purposes such as early detection of impending relapse, assessment of putative basic symptoms which might be a direct expression of the pathophysiology of the illness, and assessment of coping strategies, consensus between groups of investigators regarding assessment procedures would facilitate comparison between studies and hence help to clarify the utility of these assessments. It would be premature to conclude that existing scales have the appropriate item content and psychometric properties to justify their widespread use. However, consistency in the finding of studies using these scales suggest that they are useful instruments for clarifying the relevance of the subjective experiences of schizophrenic patients.

References

Andreasen, N.C. (1982). Negative symptoms in schizophrenia: definition and reliability. *Archives of General Psychiatry,* **39**, 784-788.

Arieti, S. (1974). "The Interpretation of Schizophrenia". 2nd Edn. Crosby Lockwood and Staples, London.

Bandura, A. (1977). Self-efficacy: towards a unifying theory of behavioural change. *Psychological Review,* **84**, 191-215.

Bartko, J.J. and Carpenter, W.T. (1976). On the methods and theory of reliability. *Journal of Nervous and Mental Diseases,* **163**, 307-312.

Bebbington, P. and Kuipers, L. (1988). Social influences on schizophrenia. *In* "Schizophrenia, the Major Issues". (Eds P. Bebbington and P. McGuffin). Heinemann Medical.

Birchwood, M., Smith, J., MacMillan, F., Hogg, B., Prasad, R., Harvey, C. and Bering, S. (1989). Predicting relapse in schizophrenia: the development and implementation of an early signs monitoring system using patients and families as observers, a preliminary investigation. *Psychological Medicine,* **19**, 649-656.

Bleuler, E. (1911). "Dementia Praecox or the Group of Schizophrenias". Translated by I. Zinkin, 1950. International University Press, New York.

Boker, W., Brenner, H.D. and Wurgler, S. (1989). Vulnerability-linked deficiencies, psychopathology and coping behaviour of schizophrenics and their relatives. *British Journal of Psychiatry,* **155**, (Suppl. 5) 128-135.

Bouricius, J.K. (1989). Negative symptoms and emotions in schizophrenia. *Schizophrenia Bulletin,* **15**, 201-207.

Breier, A. and Strauss, J.S. (1983). Self-control in psychotic disorders. *Archives of General Psychiatry,* **40**, 1141-1145.

Brett-Jones, J., Garety, P. and Hemsley, D. (1987). Measuring delusional experiences: A method and its application. *British Journal of Clinical Psychology*, **26**, 257-266.

Brewin, C.R., Veltro, F., Wing, J.K., MacCarthy, B. and Brugha, T.S. (1990). The assessment of psychiatric disability in the community: a comparison of clinical staff and family interviews. *British Journal of Psychiatry*, **157**, 671-674.

Chapman, L.J. and Chapman, J.P. (1987). The search for symptoms predictive of schizophrenia. *Schizophrenia Bulletin*, **13**, 497-503.

Cohen, C.I. and Berk, L.A. (1985). Personal coping styles of schizophrenic outpatients. *Hospital and Community Psychiatry*, **36**, 407-410.

Csikszentmihalyi, M. and Larson, R. (1987). Validity and reliability of the Experience-Sampling Methods. *Journal of Nervous and Mental Diseases*, **176**, 526-536.

Cutting, J. and Dunne, F. (1989). Subjective experience of schizophrenia. *Schizophrenia Bulletin*, **15**, 217-231.

deVries, M.W. and Delespaul, P.A.E.G. (1989). Time context and subjective experience in schizophrenic psychosis. *Schizophrenia Bulletin*, **15**, 233-244.

Doherty, J.P., Van Kammen, D.P., Siris, S.G. and Marder, S.R. (1978). Stages of onset of schizophrenic psychosis. *American Journal of Psychiatry*, **135**, 420-426.

Donlon, P.T. and Blacker, K.H. (1973). Stages of schizophrenic decompensation and reintegration. *Journal of Nervous and Mental Diseases*, **157**, 200-209.

Falloon, I.R.H. and Talbot, R.E. (1981). Persistent auditory hallucinations: coping mechanisms and implications for management. *Psychological Medicine*, **11**, 329-339.

Frith, C.D. and Done, D.J. (1988). Towards a neuropsychology of schizophrenia. *British Journal of Psychiatry*, **153**, 437-443.

Frith, C.D. and Done, D.J. (1989). Experiences of alien control in schizophrenia reflect a disorder in the central monitoring of action. *Psychological Medicine*, **19**, 359-363.

Garety, P. (1985). Delusions: problems in definition and measurement. *British Journal of Medical Psychology*, **58**, 25-34.

Gross, G. (1985). Bonner Untersuchungsinstrument zur standardiserten Erhebung und Dokumentation van Basissymptomen (BSABS). *In* "Basisstadien endogener Psychosen und das Borderline-Problems". (Ed. G. Huber), pp. 29-46. Scattauer, Stuttgart.

Heinrichs, D.W., Cohen, B.P. and Carpenter, W.T. (1985). Early insight and management of schizophrenic decompensation. *Journal of Nervous and Mental Diseases*, **173**, 133-138.

Hemsley, D.R. (1977). What have cognitive deficits to do with schizophrenic symptoms? *British Journal of Psychiatry*, **130**, 167-173.

Herz, M.I. and Melville, C. (1980). Relapse in schizophrenia. *American Journal of Psychiatry*, **137**, 801-805.

Hirsch, S.R. and Jolley, A.G. (1989). The dysphoric syndrome in schizophrenia and its implications for relapse. *British Journal of Psychiatry*, **155**, (Suppl. 5) 46-50.

Jaspers, K. (1913). "General Psychopathology". Translated by J. Hoenig and M.W. Hamilton 1959. Manchester University Press, Manchester.

Liddle, P.F. (1986). Do subjective symptoms underlie observable deficits in schizophrenia? Third Bi-annual Winter Workshop on Schizophrenia, Schaldming, Austria.

Liddle, P.F. and Barnes, T.R.E. (1988). The subjective experience of deficits in schizophrenia. *Comprehensive Psychiatry*, **29**, 157-164.

MacCarthy, B., Benson, J. and Brewin, C.R. (1986). Task motivation and problem appraisal in long-term schizophrenia. *Psychological Medicine*, **16**, 431-438.

McCandless-Glimcher, L., McKnight, S., Hamera, E., Smith, B.L., Peterson, K.A. and

Plumlee, A.A. (1986). Use of symptoms by schizophrenics to monitor and regulate their illness. *Hospital and Community Psychiatry,* **37**, 929-933.

McEvoy, J.P., Apperson, L.J., Appelbaum, P.S. Ortlip, P., Brecosky, J., Hammill, K., Geller, J.L. and Roth, L. (1989). Insight in schizophrenia. Its relationship to acute psychopathology. *Journal of Nervous and Mental Disease,* **177**, 43-47

McGlashan, T.H. (1987). Recovery style from mental illness and long-term outcome. *Journal of Nervous and Mental Disease,* **175**, 681-685.

Morley, S. (1989). Single Case research. *In* "Behavioural and Mental Health Research". (Eds G. Parry and F. Watts). A Handbook of Skills and Methods. Hove LEA.

Parker, G., Tupling, H. and Brown, L.B. (1979). A parental bonding instrument. *British Journal of Medical Psychology,* **52**, 1-10.

Petho, B. and Bitter, I. (1985). Types of complaints in psychiatric and internal medical patients. *Psychopathology,* **18**, 241-253.

Roback, H.B. and Abramowitz, S.I. (1979). Insight and hospital adjustment. *Canadian Journal of Psychiatry,* **24**, 233-236.

Scott, R.D. and Alwyn, S. (1978). Patient-parent relationships and the course and outcome of schizophrenia. *British Journal of Medical Psychology,* **51**, 343-362.

Shapiro, M.B. (1961). A method of measuring changes specific to the individual psychiatric patient. *British Journal of Medical Psychology,* **34**, 151-155.

Soskis, D.A. and Bowers, M.B. (1969). The schizophrenic experience. *Journal of Nervous and Mental Disease,* **149**, 443-449.

Strauss, J.S. (1989). Subjective experience of schizophrenia: towards a new dynamic psychiatry - II. *Schizophrenia Bulletin,* **15**, 179-187.

World Health Organization (1973). Report on the International Pilot Study of Schizophrenia. World Health Organization, Geneva.

Thurm, I. and Haefner, H. (1987). Perceived vulnerability, relapse risk and coping in schizophrenia. An explorative study. *European Archives of Psychiatry and Neurological Sciences,* **237**, 46-53.

Warner, R. and Atkinson, M. (1988). The relationship between schizophrenic patients' perceptions of their parents and the course of their illness. *British Journal of Psychiatry,* **153**, 344-353.

Zubin, J., Steinhauer, S.R., Dax, R. and Kammen, D.P. (1985). Schizophrenia at the crossroads: A blueprint for the 80s. *Comprehensive Psychiatry,* **26**, 217-240.

9. The Assessment of Suicidal Risk

Keith Hawton

Risk of suicide

The risk of suicide in patients with psychiatric disorders is considerably higher than that of the general population, the risk in those with manic-depressive and schizophrenic disorders being especially high. Before considering the instruments which are available for evaluating suicidal risk and behaviour in manic-depressive and schizophrenic disorders, some specific findings concerning suicidal risk in these two conditions will be outlined.

Manic-depressive Disorder   Two reviews of several follow-up studies of patients with affective disorders have concluded that approximately 15% end their lives by suicide (Guze and Robins, 1970; Jamison, 1986), a risk approximately 30 times that of the general population. Guze and Robins (1970) noted that the risk tends to be highest relatively early in the course of the disorder and that, in contrast with schizophrenia (see below), suicide nearly always occurs during episodes of depression rather than remission.

Specific risk factors for suicide in patients with affective disorders have been examined. In a comparison of 64 depressed suicides with 128 living individuals with depressive disorder Barraclough and Pallis (1975) found that the following characteristics were significantly more common among the suicides: male sex, older age (females only), single status, living alone, a history of suicide attempts, and symptoms of insomnia, impaired memory and self-neglect. More recent studies by Beck and colleagues have highlighted the importance of hopelessness (negative expectations about the future) as a key factor in suicide risk of depressives (Beck *et al.,* 1985, 1990).

Schizophrenia   Due to the very marked differences that used to exist regarding diagnostic criteria for schizophrenia, a situation which has only recently been more or less resolved, the risk of suicide in patients with this disorder is not altogether clear. In a review of a series of early follow-up studies Miles (1977) concluded that approximately 10% of people with schizophrenia die by suicide. With our current tighter diagnostic criteria it is possible that the risk is even higher. Miles noted that the risk is especially high during the early years of the illness.

Comparison of schizophrenic suicides with living individuals with schizophrenia indicates that those at special risk are: males, the relatively young, those with a chronic illness characterized by relapses and remissions, those with depressive symptoms and/or suicidal ideas, and the unemployed (Roy, 1982). On the basis of a further comparative study, Drake and colleagues (1984) have made the important point that suicide in schizophrenia rarely occurs during an acute psychotic episode, but usually during remission and especially when patients are feeling very pessimistic about their disorder and its implications for their future. At particular risk appear to be patients who have attained a relatively high level of education before their illness developed, subsequently retained over-ambitious (although non-delusional) expectations of themselves and yet are all too well aware of the effects of the illness on their functioning. They tend to become depressed, not so much with biological features of depression, but with psychological symptoms such as feelings of inadequacy, hopelessness and suicidal ideas.

Difficulties in prediction of suicide

Clinical experience highlights how difficult assessment of suicide risk can be. It is important to emphasize that several factors mitigate against accurate prediction of suicide, especially when assessment scales are used.

The first problem is due to suicide being (fortunately) a relatively rare event, even in high risk groups such as patients with psychotic disorders, and the crudeness of our predictors. This means that while we can probably identify the majority of patients who are at risk of eventual suicide, in doing so we will identify a vast number more who are actually not at serious risk. Thus while sensitivity of risk assessment may be high, specificity and hence overall predictive power are low.

A second problem is that, since most patients with psychoses receive treatment, risk factors which have been identified from research are in fact characteristics of patients who have killed themselves in spite of treatment. Thus they may not be so useful in assessing suicide risk in general.

A third problem is that, while in clinical practice we are usually concerned with whether patients are at risk now or in the very near future, risk factors identified from research studies are those which concern long-term risk. These are not necessarily identical with those which are associated with short-term risk.

Fourthly, most risk factors, apart from gender, are not necessarily permanent. Thus, risk in the individual patient can change, such as when a happily married woman with a satisfying job and teenage children becomes, a few years later, a disillusioned divorcee, who has been made redundant, seen her children leave home and started drinking heavily. Thus prediction of long-term risk on the basis of current factors can be misleading.

Finally, because risk factors for suicide are identified through studies of groups of patients they are not necessarily helpful with regard to assessment of an individual patient. It must be remembered that risk factors distinguish groups of patients who have killed themselves from groups who have not – this does not mean that every individual who kills himself or herself has these characteristics.

The role of specific measures in the assessment of suicide risk

Scales are available which are directly or indirectly relevant to assessment of suicide risk in patients with affective disorders. One direct measure is the Risk Estimator for Suicide (Motto *et al.*, 1985). Indirect measures include the Hope-lessness Scale (Beck *et al.*, 1974*b*) and the Scale for Suicide Ideation (Beck *et al.*, 1979). These are discussed in detail below.

There are no scales designed specifically for assessing suicide risk in patients with schizophrenia.

Of relevance to patients in both diagnostic categories who make suicide attempts are the measures which have been developed to assess degree of suicidal intent (Suicide Intent Scale), risk of repeat attempts (Risk of Repetition Scale) and of suicide (Tuckman and Youngman Scale). Only the last of these will be discussed in detail, and brief comments made about the other two.

The major use of these scales is in research studies. They should never be used as the sole or even major component of suicide risk assessment in clinical practice. While coverage of all the items in the relevant scales will help ensure that important aspects of assessment are not forgotten, this process only serves as part of the clinical assessment. The assessment must also rely on enquiry about and consideration of other more intangible factors (e.g. strength of emotional ties to family members, the trust the patient has in the clinician, possible counter-transference issues, and the likely effectiveness of treatment in the particular case). The patient's current circumstances may also be very relevant. For example, Morgan (1979) has suggested that suicide in psychiatric hospital inpatients may be associated with a process of "malignant alienation", such as when angry and provocative behaviour has led to a progressive deterioration in a patient's relationship with others, including ward staff. Misleading clinical improvement may be a further such factor (Morgan and Priest, 1984).

The Assessment Procedures

Risk Estimator for Suicide
(Motto et al., 1985)

This interviewer-rated scale was developed to assess the risk of suicide in depressed and/or suicidal patients. The items in the scale were identified from a prospective study of a large sample of psychiatric inpatients, 4.9% of whom committed suicide during a 2-year follow-up period (Motto *et al.*, 1985). It takes only a few minutes to complete the scale. Thus in a preliminary field test, volunteer crisis workers took on average 4.5 min to complete it (Motto, 1985).

The scale contains 15 items, which include demographic (e.g. age, occupation), psychosocial (e.g. financial circumstances, stress) and clinical characteristics (e.g. sleep duration, suicidal ideas), plus a single item concerning the interviewer's reaction to the patient. The items can be enquired about during a specific interview, or completed on the basis of information gathered during a routine clinical assessment. Each item is given a weighted score, and the total score is used to assess relative risk of suicide during the following 2 years.

Reliability and validity
The author is unaware of any information on reliability of the scale. Its validity must be considered doubtful since an independent field test failed to find any significant

predictive validity for it (Clark *et al.*, 1987). While the authors of that study did not think that their results necessarily invalidated the scale, their study confirmed the necessity for repeated refinement and testing in order to develop an adequate scale of this kind, a procedure which will require many years to complete, and reminds us just how far we are from finding a truly efficient predictive measure of suicide (Pokorny, 1983). It may be that the search for such a measure, for which clinicians and researchers alike would be extremely grateful, is in fact an impossible task.

Utility

While the simplicity of the scale makes it attractive, the above comments clearly indicate that it has limited usefulness. It might provide a basis for further research in this area. However, it is certainly no substitute for a broader clinical assessment of the individual patient.

Hopelessness Scale
(Beck et al., 1974)

This scale was developed to assess the degree of current pessimism or negative attitudes towards the future, especially in depressed patients. It is appropriate for teenagers and adults of all ages with psychiatric disorders, provided there is not marked intellectual impairment. This is a self-rated scale which takes most patients between 3 and 10 min to complete. Scoring takes only a minute or two, especially if a scoring template is used.

The scale contains 20 statements, each of which is rated by the patient as true or false. The statements all refer, either positively or negatively, to the future or to how things usually work out for the patient. Each of the 20 responses is scored 0 to 1; the possible range of scores therefore being from 0 to 20. There are no absolute threshold scores, although Beck *et al.* (1985) found that nearly all patients who eventually died by suicide scored 17 or more at their original assessment. Probably the most informative use of the scale in clinical practice is when serial scores over time are obtained, together with scores for depression (e.g. the Beck Depression Inventory – see below). Consistently high hopelessness scores or an abrupt increase in score should alert the clinician to a possible change in the patient's suicide risk status and the need for further clinical assessment.

Reliability and validity

No normative data are available, except from specific studies of patients in treatment trials. In a comparative study of cognitive therapy with antidepressant treatment, for example, the mean score on the scale for depressed patients at the beginning of the study was 14 (Rush *et al.*, 1982). The author is unaware of any reports of test-retest reliability of this scale. However, correlations between individual items and the total score have been shown to be satisfactory (Beck *et al.*, 1974*b*).

A comparison of patients' ratings on the scale with ratings of hopelessness made by clinicians and with scores on a self-rated semantic differential test of hopelessness demonstrated reasonable validity (Beck *et al.,* 1974*b*). The Hopelessness Scale score was also found to correlate more highly with the pessimism item on the Beck Depression Inventory than with any other item on the depression scale.

Utility

The Hopelessness Scale is acceptable to most patients, although severely agitated or retarded individuals may (as with other self-rated measures) have trouble completing it. There is some risk that patients who wish to conceal their suicidal intentions may falsify their scores on the scale.

The Hopelessness Scale has been used extensively in research investigations, including in treatment studies of depressed patients (e.g. Rush *et al.,* 1982) and in studies of suicidal behaviour. Several investigations of attempted suicide patients have shown that while suicidal intent (see below) correlates with both depression and hopelessness scores, the latter is the crucial factor and accounts for the statistical association between depression and suicidal intent (Minkoff *et al.,* 1973; Beck *et al.,* 1975; Wetzel *et al.,* 1980; Dyer and Kreitman, 1984). The association in prospective studies between high scores on the Hopelessness Scale and eventual suicide (Beck *et al.,* 1985, 1990) has already been noted. However, it must be emphasized that in those studies there were far more high scorers who did not commit suicide than did, once again highlighting the low predictive power of measures with regard to suicide prediction.

The Hopelessness Scale is useful in clinical practice, especially if employed in conjunction with a depression measure (e.g. Beck Depression Inventory). As noted above, persistent high scores, particularly if depression is improving, or an abrupt increase in score, may indicate high or increased risk of suicidal behaviour. In suicide risk assessment, special heed should also be paid to the questions on the Beck Depression Inventory (Beck *et al.,* 1961) regarding pessimism (question 2) and suicidal ideas (question 9).

Scale for Suicidal Ideation
(Beck et al., 1979)

This interviewer-rated scale was developed to measure the intensity of current suicidal ideation and is intended for use in depressed and suicidal patients, including those who have made previous suicide attempts. Completion of the scale takes between 5 and 15 min.

There are 19 items, which cover the extent of suicidal thoughts and characteristics as well as the patient's attitude towards them, the extent of any wish to die, possible desire to make an actual suicide attempt, details of any plans for an attempt, internal deterrents against an attempt, and subjective feelings of control and/or "courage" regarding a proposed attempt. The scale can be completed in a specific interview, but it can also be readily incorporated in a clinical interview. Each of the 19 items is scored 0, 1 or 2; the total range of possible scores therefore being 0-38.

Reliability and validity

No threshold scores have been published, and no standardization or normative data are available. An inter-rater reliability coefficient of 0.83 was obtained for two assessors rating the same interviews with 25 patients (Beck *et al.,* 1979). Although Beck *et al.* (1979) stated that concurrent validity of the scale was tested by comparing scores against clinical evaluations and psychological inventory scores, no results were provided. However, scores on the scale were higher in depressed patients hospitalized because of suicidal ideas than in non-hospitalized depressed patients with equivalent depression scores.

Utility

The author has no personal experience of using the scale and it has not been employed much in research, except as a dependent variable in order to allow the influence of other factors (e.g. depression and hopelessness) on suicidal thoughts to be evaluated (Wetzel, 1976; Beck *et al.,* 1979). It may prove valuable in evaluative treatment studies of depressed and suicidal patients, and could be a useful adjunct to clinical assessment of suicide risk.

Scale for Assessing Suicide Risk of Attempted Suicides – Tuckman and Youngman Scale
(Tuckman and Youngman, 1968)

This scale was developed in order to detect attempted suicide patients at greatest risk of eventual suicide. The risk of suicide following attempted suicide is high, with 1% of UK samples dying by suicide within a year and approximately 3% dying within 3-8 years (Buglass and McCulloch, 1970; Buglass and Horton, 1974; Hawton and Fagg, 1988). The risk in patients with affective or (especially) schizophrenic disorders is even higher, and, as already noted, a history of attempted suicide is a distinguishing factor between patients with such disorders who kill themselves and those who are living.

The scale was developed on the basis of a study involving several years' follow-up of 3800 suicide attempters known to the police department in Philadelphia, among whom there were 48 deaths by suicide during the follow-up period. It can be completed in a few minutes, and the questions can be incorporated within a clinical interview. The original scale contained 17 items but three should be omitted because Tuckman and Youngman's findings for these were in the opposite direction to their original predictions. The remaining 14 items cover demographic factors, health (both physical and mental), the method and circumstances of the attempt, season of the year and previous attempts. Each item is scored 0 (absent) or 1. The risk of suicide increases in proportion to the total number of items with a positive score. In their original study Tuckman and Youngman (1968) found that the suicide rate in suicide attempters who scored positively on two to five factors was 6.98 per 1000, in those who scored 6-9 it was 19.61 per 1000, and in those who scored 10-12 the rate was 60.61 per 1000.

Reliability and validity

The author is unaware of any reliability studies on this scale, but the nature of the items is such that the reliability should be very high.

As noted above, the validity of the scale was examined in the original study. However, while the increment in rates of suicide with increasing scores is impressive, one must remember that even in those scoring 10-12 on the scale, the "false-positive" rate was extremely high. Resnick and Kendra (1973) did not find the scale to be so effective in a study of patients admitted to psychiatric hospitals, although their methodology was rather unusual. Some of the items in the scale have been confirmed by other workers as distinguishing eventual suicides from survivors (e.g. Pallis *et al.*, 1982; Hawton and Fagg, 1988).

Utility

The Tuckman and Youngman scale is easy to use, although there must be some doubt whether all items are relevant to UK populations of suicide attempters referred to general hospitals. Other scales for prediction of suicide risk in attempters are available, such as the Post-attempt Risk-assessment (parasuicide) Scales (Pallis *et al.*, 1982). At present it is not clear which is the most useful, and especially which would be most appropriate for attempted suicide patients with affective or schizophrenic disorders.

Suicide Intent Scale
(Beck et al., 1974)

This scale was developed to assess the degree of suicide intent (wish to die) associated with suicide attempts. It is a 15-item interviewer-rated scale consisting of two parts. The first part, of eight items, concerns the objective circumstances of the attempt. The second part of seven items concerns the patient's self-report about the attempt and its purpose. It takes about 10 min to complete and the questions can be readily incorporated into a clinical interview. Each item is scored 0-2; the range of scores being 0-30. A manual providing guidelines for scoring is available. There are no normative data, but experience indicates that the mean score on the scale for randomly selected suicide attempters is approximately 9.

Reliability and validity

The inter-rater reliability coefficient of the scale was 0.95 for 45 cases (Beck *et al.*, 1974*a*) and scores on the first part of the scale were significantly higher in completed suicides than in surviving attempters (Beck *et al.*, 1974*c*). Preliminary evidence is available that scores on this scale correlate with risk of eventual suicide (Pierce, 1981).

Validity

The Suicide Intent Scale is useful both in research and clinical work. New raters need to get experience and supervision in its use, because they tend to over-rate patients initially and give them too high scores. Familiarity with the manual is important. In clinical practice this scale can be an extremely useful adjunct to overall clinical asssessment.

Risk of Repetition Scale
(Buglass and Horton, 1974)

This is a simple 6-item interviewer-rated scale developed to identify degree of risk of repetition of suicide attempts. The background research was elaborate and consisted of construction of the scale on the basis of characteristics which distinguished subsequent repeaters from non-repeaters in a large cohort of attempters, followed by retesting and validation on two further large cohorts. Four items are straightforward (previous inpatient psychiatric treatment, previous outpatient psychiatric treatment, previous parasuicide (suicide attempt) resulting in general hospital admission, and not living with a relative). However, the remaining two (sociopathy and problems in the use of alcohol), although briefly defined, are likely to cause some disagreement. The author is unaware of any data on reliability of the scale.

One point is allocated for each item which is positive. Total scores range therefore from 0 - 6, the higher the score the greater the risk of repetition. In the original study 48% of patients with scores of 5 or 6 repeated attempts within a year. Other workers, including the author (Hawton, 1979), have reported similar findings.

Utility
The main use of the Risk of Repetition Scale is in research, such as when defining groups of patients for descriptive or treatment studies. While the scale can be used to assist routine clinical assessment, it would be unwise to rely solely on it in assessing risk of repetition in the individual patient.

Conclusions

It must be acknowledged that assessment instruments are only of limited value with regard to suicidal behaviour in patients with psychotic disorders. One of the main problems is the low predictive power of instruments used to assess risk of suicide. It may well be that the development of a powerful instrument for this purpose is not feasible. However, scales that are available can be helpful additions to clinical assessment. They are rather more useful in research investigations, especially when subgrouping of patients is desired, and particularly with regard to prospective follow-up studies.

References

Barraclough, B. and Pallis, D.J. (1975). Depression followed by suicide: a comparison of depressed suicides with living depressives. *Psychological Medicine, 5*, 55-61.

Beck, A.T., Ward, C.H. and Mendelson, M. (1961). An inventory for measuring depression. *Archives of General Psychiatry, 4*, 561-571.

Beck, A.T., Schuyler, D. and Herman, J. (1974a). Development of suicidal intent scales. *In* "The Prediction of Suicide". (Eds A.T. Beck., H.L.P. Resnick and D.J. Lettieri). Charles Press, Maryland.

Beck, A.T., Weissman, A., Lester, D. and Trexler, L. (1974b). The measurement of pessimism: the Hopelessness Scale. *Journal of Consulting and Clinical Psychology, 42*, 861-865.

Beck, R.W., Morris, J.B. and Beck, A.T. (1974c). Cross-validation of the Suicidal Intent Scale. *Psychological Reports, 34*, 445-446.

Beck, A.T., Kovacs, M. and Weissman, A. (1975). Hopelessness and suicidal behaviour: an overview. *Journal of the American Medical Association, 234*, 1146-1149.

Beck, A.T., Kovacs, M. and Weissman, A. (1979). Assessment of suicidal intention: the Scale for Suicide Ideation. *Journal of Consulting and Clinical Psychology, 47*, 343-352.

Beck A.T., Steer, R.A., Kovacs, M. and Garrison, B. (1985). Hopelessness and eventual suicide: a 10 year prospective study of patients hospitalised with suicidal ideation. *American Journal of Psychiatry, 145*, 559-563.

Beck, A.T., Brown, G. , Berchick, R.J., Stewart, B.L. and Steer, R.A. (1990). Relationship between hopelessness and ultimate suicide: a replication with psychiatric outpatients. *American Journal of Psychiatry, 147*, 190-195.

Buglass, D. and Horton, J. (1974). A scale for predicting subsequent suicidal behaviour. *British Journal of Psychiatry, 124*, 573-758.

Buglass, D. and McCulloch, J.W. (1970). Further suicidal behaviour: the development and validation of predictive scales. *British Journal of Psychiatry, 116*, 483-491.

Clarke, D.C., Young, M.A., Scheftner, W.A., Fawcett, J. and Fogg, L. (1987). A field test of Motto's Risk Estimator for Suicide. *American Journal of Psychiatry, 144*, 923-926.

Drake, R.E., Gates, C., Cotton, P.G. and Whitaker, A. (1984). Suicide among schizophrenics: who is at risk? *Journal of Nervous and Mental Disease, 172*, 613-617.

Dyer, J.A.T. and Kreitman, N. (1984). Hopelessness, depression and suicidal intent in parasuicide. *British Journal of Psychitary, 144*, 127-133.

Guze, S.B. and Robins, E. (1970). Suicide among primary affective disorders. *British Journal of Psychiatry, 117*, 437-438.

Hawton, K. (1979). "Evaluation of Short-term Psychiatric Intervention following Acts of Self-poisoning". Unpublished DM thesis, University of Oxford.

Hawton, K. and Fagg, J. (1988). Suicide and other causes of death following attempted suicide. *British Journal of Psychiatry, 152*, 359-366.

Jamison, K.R. (1986). Suicide and bipolar disorders. *In* "Psychobiology of Suicidal Behavior". (Eds J.J. Mann and M. Stanley). *Annals of the New York Academy of Sciences, 487*, 301-315. New York Academy of Sciences, New York.

Miles, C.P. (1977). Conditions predisposing to suicide: a review. *Journal of Nervous and Mental Disease, 164*, 231-246.

Minkoff, K., Bergmann, E., Beck, A.T. and Beck, R. (1973). Hopelessness, depression and attempted suicide. *American Journal of Psychiatry, 130*, 455-459.

Morgan, H.G. (1979). "Death Wishes: The Understanding and Management of Deliberate Self-harm". Wiley, Chichester.

Morgan, H.G. and Priest, P. (1984). Assessment of suicide risk in psychiatric in-patients. *British Journal of Psychiatry,* **145**, 467-469.

Motto, J.A. (1985). Preliminary field-testing of a Risk Estimator for Suicide. *Suicide and Life Threatening Behaviour,* **15**, 139-150.

Motto, J.A., Heilbron, D.C. and Juster, J.P. (1985). Development of a clinical instrument to estimate suicide risk. *American Journal of Psychiatry,* **142**, 680-686.

Pallis, D.J., Barraclough, B.M., Levey, A.B., Jenkins, J.S. and Sainsbury, P. (1982). Estimating suicide risk among attempted suicides: I. The development of new clinical scales. *British Journal of Psychiatry,* **141**, 37-44.

Pierce, D.W. (1981). The predictive validation of a suicidal intent scale: a five year follow-up. *British Journal of Psychiatry,* **139**, 391-396.

Pokorny, A.D. (1983). Prediction of suicide in psychiatric patients: report of a prospective study. *Archives of General Psychiatry,* **40**, 249-257.

Resnick, J.H. and Kendra, J.M. (1973). Predictive value of the "Scale for Assessing Suicide Risk" (SASR) with hospitalised psychiatric patients. *Journal of Clinical Psychology,* **29**, 187-190.

Roy, A. (1982). Suicide in chronic schizophrenia. *British Journal of Psychiatry,* **141**, 171-177.

Rush, J., Beck, A.T., Kovacs, M., Weissenburger, J. and Hollon, S.T. (1982). Comparison of the effects of cognitive therapy and pharmacotherapy on hopelessness and self-concept. *American Journal of Psychiatry,* **139**, 862-866.

Tuckman, J. and Youngman, W.F. (1968). A scale for assessing suicide risk of attempted suicides. *Journal of Clinical Psychology,* **24**, 17-19.

Wetzel, R.D. (1976). Hopelessness, depression and suicide intent. *Archives of General Psychiatry,* **33**, 1069-1073.

Wetzel, R.D., Marguiles, T., Davis, R. and Karam, E. (1980). Hopelessness, depression and suicidal intent. *Journal of Clinical Psychiatry,* **41**, 159-160.

10. The Assessment of Social Behaviour

Christos Pantelis and David A. Curson

The social behaviour of mental patients and the psychically abnormal is not at all uniform nor can it be reduced to any simple formula. Even where the form of the disorder is the same, individuals behave quite differently. A very distracted person affected by a disease-process may still maintain lively social relationships while someone suffering from a personality disorder may shut himself off from all human society and conclude his vegetative existence in complete isolation. But the majority of individuals whom we regard as psychically abnormal are also abnormal in their social behaviour. It has even been tried to make this latter a criterion for illness. The vast majority of psychically abnormal people are asocial but relatively few of them are anti-social (Karl Jaspers, 1959).

Impairments of social functioning are commonly seen in patients with schizophrenia and the psychoses. Indeed such disabilities may be prodromal symptoms, signalling the onset of the disorder, they may accompany the acute illness, or they may remain as chronic disabilities following remission of an acute psychosis (Wing, 1980). Diagnostic criteria, such as DSM-III-R (American Psychiatric Association, 1987), include such impairments of social functioning in their definition of the active, prodromal and residual phases of schizophrenia.

The need to measure social impairments or disabilities partly results from the changes in psychiatry over the last 40 years, from custodial care in chronic long-stay wards towards community-based care. Whereas previously there was a tendency to assume that length of stay could be taken as a measure of schizophrenic impairment (Wing, 1980), this was clearly inadequate in defining the disabilities and needs of these people, or in measuring change as a consequence of medical or social intervention. Consequently, scales have emerged to assess the presence and severity of psychotic symptoms as well as to measure the behavioural and other disturbances of social functioning. An important consideration in deciding between various scales is the purpose for which they will be used and the growing need for such scales to be valid and reliable in a number of settings both within and outside hospital (e.g. Brewin et al., 1990). The use of established scales allows for the replication of a study by other investigators.

Impairments in the capacity to function within a social context cover a number of different but related disabilities, which are not always clearly separable, and indeed may interact dynamically with each other as well as with the symptoms of psychosis. Because the relative independence of the various components of social impairment, or "social disablement" (Wing, 1989), and of these and psychotic symptoms is unclear, it is important to quantify the various types of impairments which come under the rubric of impaired social functioning separately and accurately (Weissman, 1975), though in practice this often poses a number of difficulties (Brugha, 1989). This chapter will focus specifically on the measurement of disturbances in social behaviour in psychotic patients.

The specific behavioural disturbances, such as overactivity, slowness, laughing or talking to self, need to be distinguished from impairments such as the more general "deficiencies" in social performance, that is, the failure to fulfil certain social roles, such as, housewife, parent, sexual partner and companion (Platt, 1986; see Chapter 11). Other aspects of impaired social functioning which need to be distinguished from impairments of behaviour include deficits in the activities of daily living, impaired social skills, disturbance of social supports/networks (Brugha, 1989), as well as burden on the family (Platt, 1985). Though aggressive behaviour is often included in scales measuring behaviour, separate scales have emerged specifically to measure violence and aggression in patients with psychosis (see Chapter 14).

In general, abnormal social behaviour can be divided into two main categories. First, a reduction or absence of socially appropriate behaviours and secondly, behaviours which are excessive and/or socially inappropriate. The former have been found to correlate with "social withdrawal", the latter with "socially embarrassing behaviour" (Wing, 1961). Behaviours in either category may have adverse effects for the individual as well as on those around them, be subject to spontaneous change over time, and change in response to social or pharmacological intervention, be it therapeutic or otherwise.

There are a number of reasons why social behaviour and its measurement is important. Social behaviour may be as clinically relevant as psychiatric symptomatology in determining response to treatment and successful rehabilitation, especially where therapeutic endeavour is aimed at maintaining the patient's links with the "real world" outside the hospital. Impairments of social behaviour may be important determinants of the degree to which families, other carers or even neighbours may tolerate individual patients. For instance, a patient with intermittent outbursts of aggression despite an excellent level of functioning in all other areas will be difficult to place compared with a patient who is continually hallucinated but withdrawn. Barnes *et al.* (1983) found that disturbed behaviours were associated with a relatively high level of distress in the patients' relatives and friends. Similarly, Gubman *et al.* (1987) found that behavioural problems were the best predictors of complaints from both family households and other types of residential care, while complaints about disturbances in social role performance were unique to family households. Also, social behaviours, such as difficulty with self-care, may influence physical health or the capacity to maintain independent living, whether or not other social performance deficits are also present. The assessment of behaviour may provide a more sensitive measure of change than other measures, such as social role performance, as a consequence of some change in the patients' circumstances or as a result of treatment. Thus, whereas the ability to fulfil his/her role as a father/mother, etc. may not alter, subtle changes in severe behavioural disturbances may provide the only evidence of the efficacy or detrimental effects of treatment, rehabilitation or other intervention. In understanding the relationship and interdependence of the various components of social functioning, it is necessary to measure these separately. Thus, impairment in social role performance, such as relationships with others, may be consequent on disturbances in social behaviour (e.g. Stevens, 1972). Finally, assessment of social behaviour and other aspects of social functioning will help in defining services to meet people's needs (Wing, 1989).

The Process of Assessment

Most social behaviour scales derive information about the patient's social functioning from the patient or from the patient's significant others. While the patient is usually the most direct and available source of information, patients with psychotic illnesses tend to underreport their disabilities (Prusoff et al., 1972; Stevens, 1972). They are also likely not to complete the interview and may show limited understanding of its purpose (Spitzer and Endicott, 1973). An informant-based interview has considerable advantages in assessing the behavioural disturbances of such patients and the information obtained in this way has been shown to be reliable and valid (Wykes and Sturt, 1986; Remington and Tyrer, 1979; Ellsworth et al., 1968; Katz and Lyerly, 1963).

Mail questionnaires and telephone interviews tend to produce a poor response rate and data of dubious reliability and validity. The self report inventory whilst being an economic method of data collection is often not appropriate for psychotic patients who are likely to be too disturbed to understand the questions or to report accurately on their social functioning. The standardized personal interview usually obtains the most complete and valid information since the interviewer can probe for more details and check on inconsistencies in responses. The semistructured interview with defined items, fixed probe questions and precoded ratings allows the interviewer freedom to make additional probes in order to make a final rating and is the most recommended method for gathering data on social behaviour (Platt, 1986). An appropriate scale for the assessment of social behaviour needs to cover a broad range of observable behaviours, and should also possess demonstrated reliability, validity, sensitivity to change, and a well developed quantitative scoring system. In addition, adequate inter-rater reliability must be confirmed in each new study or throughout the assessment period. It should be relatively easy to administer in a reasonable time and it should have acquired some degree of acceptance in the field, because of its proven "track record".

Several rating scales used for the measurement of psychiatric symptoms have sections for "observed" ratings, which include behavioural items. Examples include the Present State Examination (Wing et al., 1974), Inpatient Multidimensional Psychiatric Scale (IMPS) (Lorr and Klett, 1967), Comprehensive Psychopathological Rating Scale (CPRS) (Asberg *et al.*, 1978), Brief Psychiatric Rating Scale (BPRS) (Overall and Gorham, 1962), the Manchester Scale (Krawiecka *et al.*, 1977) and the Scale for the Assessment of Negative Symptoms (Andreasen, 1982). However, the range of behaviours covered in such scales is generally too narrow and the ratings are based on interviews with the patient during the period of the interview only, with the attendant drawbacks described above.

A number of scales designed specifically for the purpose of assessing the social functioning of psychotic patients have tended to mix aspects of social behaviour with items assessing social role performance. Indeed, there is considerable overlap between these. Wing (1989) in discussing the distinction between two schedules, one measuring behavioural impairments and the other for role performance considers that the main distinction between them is "that the latter kind measures higher level skills and is much less relevant to the problems of severely disabled people who can perform very few social roles". Wallace (1986) provides a review of many of these instruments, some of which do provide adequate coverage of behavioural items; these include the Katz Adjustment Scale (Katz and Lyerly, 1963), the Psychiatric Status Schedule (Spitzer *et al.*, 1970), the Psychiatric Evaluation Form (Endicott and Spitzer, 1972*a*), the Current and Past Psychopathology Scale (Endicott and Spitzer, 1972*b*) and the Nurses Observation Scale for Inpatient Evaluation (NOSIE-30) (Honigfeld *et al.*, 1966). Rosen *et al.* (1989) have reviewed a number of other scales developed more recently, or which were not covered in detail by Wallace (1986). These include some of the scales discussed below, as well as scales such as the Disability Assessment Scale (Schubart *et al.*, 1986) developed by the World Health Organisation, and scales providing global measures of functioning, such as the Global Assessment Scale (Endicott *et al.*, 1976). As before, a number of these schedules tend to mix behavioural disturbances with items covering impairments of social role performance, while scales providing a global assessment do not allow distinction between symptoms or aspects of more general functioning (Rosen *et al.*, 1989). The WHO Disability Assessment Scale (WHO/DAS 1988; Schubart *et al.*, 1986) incorporates the Ward Behaviour Schedule, discussed below as well as other scales derived from the MRC Social Psychiatry Unit (Wing, 1989)(see Chapters 1, 2, 3, 5 and 6 for above scales).

In this chapter we review five rating scales in detail which most closely approximate to the desired criteria discussed above, and which allow behavioural items to be scored separately from other impairments of social functioning: The Ward Behaviour Scale (Wing, 1961), The Social Behaviour Assessment Schedule (Platt *et al.*, 1978, 1980, 1983), The Social Behaviour Schedule (Wykes and Sturt, 1986; Sturt and Wykes, 1987) and the Current Behavioural Schedule (Owens and Johnstone 1980; Johnstone *et al.*, 1981, 1985). The last two instruments have been developed from the Ward Behaviour Scale. The fifth assessment instrument is a relatively new rating scale, The Life Skills Profile (Rosen *et al.*, 1989).

Other instruments such as the Rehabilitation Evaluation of Hall and Baker (REHAB) (Baker and Hall, 1983), are covered in the chapter on assessment of social functioning and dependency (Stayte and Pugh, this volume), which should be read together with this chapter. Readers are also referred to the comprehensive review by Wallace (1986) for details of some of the other schedules mentioned above.

The Assessment Procedures

Ward Behaviour Scale (WBS)
(Wing, J.K., 1961)

The Ward Behaviour Scale was derived from a behaviour rating scale constructed for the purpose of measuring change in the behaviour of moderately handicapped male schizophrenic patients during courses of rehabilitation. Principal components analysis revealed two factors representing "social withdrawal" and "socially embarrassing behaviour". Both were consistent and reliable and the scores differentiated significantly between three clinical subgroups of patients (Wing, 1961). The final and simpler 12-item scale was constructed because of its suitability for all grades of schizophrenic patient and could be administered on a large scale. It was used to test the validity of a simple subclassification of schizophrenia based on features of the mental state of the patient.

The original scale was designed for use in patients with chronic schizophrenia who were resident for long periods in hospital (Wing, 1989; Curson *et al.*, 1992). It was later expanded to include non-psychotic items, this version (the Patient Behaviour Schedule) being used to investigate the "new" long-stay, which included patients with conditions other than schizophrenia (Mann and Cree, 1976; Mann and Sproule, 1972). The original scale has also been used in community surveys of patients with schizophrenia (McCreadie, 1982, 1990).

The scale is administered by nursing staff or other informants who know the patient well. It takes 10 to 15 min to administer. The staff can rate by ticking boxes adjacent to descriptions of behaviour which best describe the patient's behaviour during the previous week. The scale may also be completed by interviewing the key informant. The 12 items are: slowness of movement, underactivity, overactivity, conversation, social withdrawal, leisure interests, laughing and talking to self, posturing and mannerisms, threatening or violent behaviour, personal hygiene (incontinence), personal appearance, and behaviour at meal times.

Scoring for each item is on a three-point scale (0 to 2) representing increasing severity of the behavioural disturbance from absent to severe. Because of the limited range of scoring, the threshold for scoring above zero on any item is generally high. The behaviour has to be extreme or marked but not necessarily continuous. For example, the item for underactivity:

rate 2 – stood or sat in one place all the time, with little movement and even with encouragement was very difficult to get moving.

rate 1 – showed periods of extreme underactivity as in (2) but at other times was not underactive.

rate 0 – showed no underactivity.

As described above, factor analysis revealed two subtotals representing "Social Withdrawal" (SW) and "Socially Embarrassing Behaviour" (SE) (Wing, 1961). Items which contribute to the SE score (maximum 8) are: overactivity, talking to self, mannerisms, and threats of violence. The remainder give the SW score (maximum 16). Total WBS score and the two subscores provide useful summary measures. However, scores for individual items may also provide useful information.

Reliability and validity
The WBS is a valid and reliable measure of disturbed social behaviour in patients with chronic schizophrenia. Inter-rater, inter-informant and test-retest reliability data were published nearly 30 years ago (Wing, 1961); the SW score showed good inter-rater agreement (0.72 to 0.91) and was reliable over time (0.61 to 0.90), whereas the SE score was less reliably rated (inter-rater agreement: 0.36 to 0.80; reliability over time: 0.16 to 0.93). The relationship of the behavioural ratings and symptoms was assessed by comparison with clinical classification based on the patient's mental state (Wing, 1961).

Utility
The WBS is one of the earliest instruments for reliably measuring social behaviour in psychotic patients. It has been used in numerous studies of schizophrenia (e.g. Wing, 1961; Wing and Brown, 1970; McCreadie, 1982; Curson et al., 1992) and two of the other scales below have been derived from it (Social Behaviour Schedule and the Current Behavioural Schedule). Its two subscores, SW and SE, are particularly useful since they are separate measures of the behavioural components of "negative" and "positive" psychotic symptoms. The SW items embrace many of the features of the schizophrenic "defect state". It can be administered rapidly, thus allowing large numbers of patients to be assessed readily. Its two principal shortcomings are that while ensuring reliability the high threshold for rating any abnormality makes it an inappropriate instrument for assessing mild behavioural disturbance and, for the same reason, it is a relatively insensitive instrument for measuring change.

The Social Behaviour Schedule (SBS)
(Wykes and Sturt, 1986, 1987)

The SBS has been developed alongside a separate but complementary schedule assessing role performance, the Social Role Performance Schedule (see Chapter 11 this volume and Wing, 1989). It provides a measure of 21 behavioural problems and is based on work by Wing (1961) and Wing and Brown (1970) with chronic institutionalized populations. The items of the Schedule are those that might be expected to lead to a subject being admitted to a day or residential facility as they would tend to interfere with daily life and/or disturb family or neighbours. More recently, a shortened version of this scale has been developed for use together with a new instrument, the MRC Needs for Care Assessment (Brewin *et al.*, 1987; Wing, 1989).

The schedule has been used in long-stay populations (Mann and Cree, 1976; Mann and Sproule, 1972; Wykes, 1982), hostel populations (Hewett *et al.*, 1975; Ryan and Wing, 1979) and more recently in community studies (Wykes *et al.*, 1982; Campbell *et al.*, 1990). It takes 15 to 30 min to administer.

The scale requires a trained interviewer who discusses each item with a key informant, either a relative or key member of the patient's caring staff, such as a charge nurse or day centre or hostel supervisor, who has been familiar with the patient over the previous month. Twenty specific behavioural items are rated with scores reflecting the severity of the behavioural disturbance. The items are: little spontaneous communication, incoherence of speech, odd or inappropriate conversation, inappropriate social mixing, hostility, demanding attention, suicidal ideas or behaviour, panic attacks or phobias, overactivity or restlessness, laughing or talking to self, acting out bizarre ideas, posturing and mannerisms, socially unacceptable habits, destructive behaviour, depression, inappropriate sexual behaviour, poor self care, slowness, underactivity, and poor attention span. There is an additional item, "other behaviour", which allows for ratings of behavioural problems not itemized on the schedule. The latter has included a number of behaviours, such as problems with alcohol, eating, poor memory, etc. which do not occur frequently. These behavioural items are followed by questions on work, leisure activities, aims for the future and presence of physical or other disabilities. Most of the items are rated on a five-point scale (0 to 4). A zero indicates acceptable behaviour and a score of 1 on any item is considered to be within the limits of normality. Pathological scores are therefore between 2 and 4, with scores of 3 and 4 indicating severe disturbances of behaviour.

Two scores derived from the 21 items are the "mild and severe problems score" (BSM or Behaviour Score Moderate) obtained by counting the number of items scoring 2 or more, and the "severe behaviour problems score" (BSS or Behaviour Score Severe) which is the number of behaviours scored as 3 or more.

Reliability and validity
The reliability of this schedule is high and these data have been presented by Wykes and Sturt (1986): inter-rater agreement of 84-100%; inter-informant agreement of 70-90%; a test-retest agreement of 72-96%; inter-setting agreement of 71-97%.

Data for the validity of the schedule have not yet been presented by the authors. However, MacCarthy *et al.* (1991) and Pantelis *et al.* (1991), have examined the factor structure of the SBS. By identifying only those (nine) items from the SBS considered to reflect the behavioural equivalents of the three syndromes in schizophrenia (Liddle, 1987) three factors were derived which appeared to resemble these three syndromes in schizophrenia. Using factor scores derived from the Manchester scale (Krawiecka *et al.*, 1977), Pantelis *et al.* (1991) have found high correlations between these syndromes and the factor scores derived from these nine SBS items.

Utility

The SBS is a very useful instrument covering a broad range of problem behaviours commonly encountered in psychiatric patients. It is relatively brief in duration and is reliable, though training is required to achieve high levels of inter-rater agreement. Some of the probe questions are poorly worded and some of the anchor point definitions for scoring are similarly imprecise. It is generally considered to be sensitive to change, though Rosen *et al.* (1989) consider that some of its sensitivity may have been sacrificed in favour of test-retest reliability. It can be used in a residential or community setting.

We have encountered some other problems with the SBS. For some of the items the scoring does not reflect a smooth gradation in severity. For example, on the item "taking the initiative with communication" many patients may differ quite widely but have to be given a score of "1" because this problem behaviour was not severe enough for a score of "2". There is no specific item for rating social withdrawal, though this was included in the original WBS (see above). If a patient is not interested in making social contacts with others he is rated as "0" on the item for "social mixing", which is clearly inappropriate as this places him with patients who are mixing normally. The item for "other behaviours" needs to be considered carefully and it is best to make a detailed note of the inappropriate behaviour on the form to assist in later analysis. In the South Camden survey (Campbell *et al.*, 1990), for instance, suspiciousness was found to be a problem in a significant proportion of those patients identified in the community, necessitating a rating under the item for "other behaviours". For this group of patients it would have been particularly interesting to rate this item separately, as they proved to be a difficult group to interview. Finally, for the item on "leisure activities", patients sometimes qualify for rating in more than one category. A patient may be scored as "2" if he has passive leisure interests, even if he is otherwise unresponsive to attempts to engage him in other activities which would be rated as "3" or "4". Despite these criticisms, the SBS is a useful and informative scale for use in this population.

Social Behaviour Assessment Schedule (SBAS)
(Platt et al., 1978, 1980 and 1983)

The SBAS was designed to provide a comprehensive assessment of behaviour and social role performance in relation to some independent variable causing change, such as severity of illness or treatment, and to assess the impact of these measures on the patient and his or her significant others. Social behaviour is covered in section B of this comprehensive schedule.

The schedule has been used in schizophrenic outpatients (Curson *et al.*, 1985; Gibbons *et al.*, 1984) including a randomized control trial of maintenance antipsychotic therapy (Barnes *et al.*, 1983), acute psychiatric inpatients (Hirsch *et al.*, 1979) and the families of alcoholic women in Germany (Lutz *et al.*, 1980). It takes 60 to 90 min to administer the full schedule, whilst Section B (patient behaviour) takes approximately 15 to 30 min.

There is a comprehensive training manual and rating guide. The full schedule consists of six sections A to F. Section A contains 22 questions about demographic characteristics of the patient, the household, and the significant other.

Section B contains 66 questions assessing the severity, time of onset, and distress experienced by the significant other of 22 patient behaviours. Section C includes 48 items covering social role performance, changes in that performance and when it changed, and distress to the significant other caused by problems in these areas. Section D covers 104 questions about the conditions in the household, changes in conditions and effects of such change on patient and significant other. Section E covers 11 stressful life events and their effect on the patient's illness. Section F contains 23 questions about assistance received from others outside the household, including relatives and helping agencies.

The schedule has been designed as a standardized, semistructured interview with the patient's most closely involved relative or friend. Though it can also be administered to professional health care workers, items about informant's distress and the section on informant's support may have to be omitted, as they will be less relevant in this setting. The schedule covers a period of 1 month before the interview.

The Social Behaviour section (Section B) covers 22 "behaviours" which are commonly associated with psychiatric disorders, including the psychoses. These are: misery, withdrawal, slowness, forgetfulness, underactivity, overdependence, indecisiveness, worrying, fearfulness, obsessionality, odd ideas, overactivity, unpredictability, irritability, rudeness, violence, parasuicide, offensive behaviour, heavy drinking, self-neglect, complaints about bodily aches and pains, and odd behaviour. No attempt is made to rate clinical symptoms or to use clinical categories.

Three ratings are made for each behaviour item. The first is an evaluation of the presence or absence of the particular behaviour; severity is rated on a three-point scale (0 to 2). The second rating relates to onset of the behaviour, i.e. when the reported behaviour was first observed by the informant. The third rating provides a measure of informant's distress in response to the reported behaviour using a four-point scale (0 to 3); scores of 1 and 2 indicate an increasing level of distress, while a 3 rating is given for "resignation" when the informant no longer reports emotional distress and has become accustomed to the behaviour over time. In the study by Barnes *et al.* (1983) the addition of ratings for an informant response of "resignation" with a score equivalent to "moderate distress", almost doubled the mean informant distress scores in the population studied, indicating how important resignation is as a measure of burden. The scores on the six sections are combined to give patient scores for disturbed behaviour, role performance, and objective burden. Scores are derived relating to burden on the significant other resulting from the disturbed behaviour or impairment in social performance. Another technique for interpreting the data is to itemize those behaviours in rank order of prevalence occurring in more than 25 per cent of the sample. In this way assessments over time may reveal changes in prevalence and patterns of disturbed behaviours with any attendant changes in informant distress. It also permits the identification of types of behaviour provoking the most distress, for example, behaviours associated with "negative" psychotic symptoms rather than "positive" ones.

Reliability and validity
Full details of the rationale, development, structure and reliability of the instrument can be found in Platt *et al.* (1980). The inter-rater reliabilities for some of the items of the initial version of the scale were low. However, the scale has been modified with improvement in these reliabilities. Inter-rater reliabilities for total scores are above 0.9, and above 0.7 for most of the individual items.

Utility
One of us (DAC), has extensive experience of the SBAS, having been involved in two of the early studies in which it was used (Curson *et al.*, 1985; Barnes *et al.*, 1983). The full schedule is time consuming but with adequate interviewing skills informants, especially relatives, do not find it laborious. It provides a comprehensive assessment of the patient's social life and is sensitive to change (Platt *et al.*, 1981). In the study by Curson *et al.* (1985) the SBAS detected early schizophrenic relapse in some patients several weeks before a clinical relapse became apparent. It has also been used to assess differences between outcome for patients receiving short versus long hospitalization (Hirsch *et al.*, 1979).

The patient behaviour section could be used for psychotic long-stay inpatients as an alternative to the SBS, although the range for rating severity is narrower and the threshold for rating a behaviour as present is higher. The full SBAS is excellent for use in schizophrenic outpatients living with their families and adds an additional dimension to social behaviour by having items assessing the impact of behaviour on those close to the patient (i.e. distress and burden). The full instrument is not appropriate for use in long stay hospital inpatients because of the limited opportunity for such patients to perform social roles and because of the difference in the nature of the relationship with professional mental health workers compared with relatives or others living in a household.

Current Behavioural Schedule (CBS)
(Johnstone, E. C. et al., 1980, 1981 and 1985)

The CBS was developed by the Northwick Park Group in the late 1970s. As well as a scale describing the behavioural impairments of patients, these researchers required a schedule which would assess the opinion of those constantly with the patient about the presence of various psychopathological features. It is derived partly from the Ward Behaviour Scale of Wing (1961).

It has been employed in studies of patients with chronic schizophrenia and manic depressive psychosis on the long stay wards of a mental hospital (Owens and Johnstone, 1980; Johnstone *et al.*, 1985). It has also proved useful in the assessment of patients with chronic schizophrenia discharged from such wards into the community (Johnstone *et al.*, 1981, 1984). The schedule takes 15 to 30 min to administer. Information is obtained by interviewing an informant, such as a nurse or relative, who has had close contact with the patient and can provide a description of behaviour over the previous 6 months.

The schedule is divided into eight sections: Section A covers social behaviour: spontaneous contacts, response to approaches, ability to carry out instructions, general social behaviour such as table manners, dressing and cleanliness, appearance, and social withdrawal; Section B covers activities: employment, leisure activities, general level of activity, nature of activity; Section C rates overactivity; Section D is for exhibited abnormal behaviour: laughing or muttering to self, hallucinations, delusions, posturing and mannerisms, obsessional activities, incoherence of speech; Section E records antisocial acts: antisocial behaviour and uncontrolled aggressive outbursts; Section F rates incontinence; Section G assesses stability of behaviour; and Section H covers current medication and difficulties with compliance.

The scoring for most of the items in each section is on a three-point scale (0 to 2); a score of "0" represents severe, "1" indicates moderate in severity and/or frequency and "2" represents absent. Scoring for employment in the activity section is on a five-point scale (0 to 4); for antisocial acts scores are from "0 to 3"; incontinence is also rated on a four-point scale (0 to 3). The item scores for this schedule are summed to give a maximum attainable score of 50. A score of 50 is indicative of "a very basic level of performance" (Owens and Johnstone, 1980). The lower the score, the more abnormal is the patient. Subscores can be derived for each section and used in comparative analysis as discussed below.

Reliability and validity

The schedule has been derived from the Ward Behaviour Schedule (Wing, 1961). Inter-rater agreement achieved by the two authors for the total scores and the sub-scores ranged from 0.98 to 1.0. There were very significant relationships between negative features of schizophrenia, cognitive functioning, neurological variables and behavioural performance, although there was no significant relationship between positive features of schizophrenia and any of these four abnormalities (Owens and Johnstone, 1980). Unfortunately, the authors did not provide correlation coefficients but only the levels of significance, although these appear to be acceptable (range $p < 0.02$ to $p < 0.001$).

Utility

The CBS proved to be sensitive and reliable when used to assess patients with chronic schizophrenia (Johnstone *et al.*, 1981, 1984). In the comparison of inpatient manic-depressives, inpatient schizophrenics, and discharged schizophrenics the three groups had total scores on the CBS which did not significantly differ, but the authors note that the scale is composed of a number of elements which may not relate to one another (Johnstone *et al.*, 1985). The elements giving rise to the abnormality in the total CBS score did appear to differ between the groups. When the differences in age and length of illness were taken into account, it was found that there was very little difference between the schizophrenic outpatients and inpatients, but there were significant differences between manic depressive and schizophrenic patients on a majority of items. The manic depressives showed less exhibited abnormal behaviour but more overactivity, antisocial acts, incontinence, and instability of their condition. It would seem, therefore, that section subscores may be more informative than simply using the CBS total score when comparing different psychotic populations in either cross-sectional surveys or when monitoring behaviour change over time.

The Life Skills Profile (LSP)
(Rosen et al., 1989)

This is a recently developed scale, devised to assess reliably and validly those aspects of social functioning that affect survival and adaptation in the community. It has been devised from a need to study the effects of transferring patients from hospital to community (Rosen *et al.*, 1989). It includes 39 items which were derived from a much larger number covering specific behaviours and living skills. The impact or burden on the rater is also assessed. The LPS has been developed in patients suffering with schizophrenia in hospital and also in a variety of settings outside hospital, such as family home, boarding houses, hostels, and psychiatrically staffed community facilities (Rosen *et al.*, 1989). It takes 15 to 30 min to administer.

The scoring sheet is relatively easy to use, requiring the rater to circle the appropriate response and the items are clearly laid out. The scale is designed for use by an informant who knows the patient well. A trained interviewer is not required. The scale is designed to assess an individual's general functioning during the previous 6 months. It has not been designed to assess functioning during periods of crisis or illness, and has been developed to assess patients' functioning during periods of stability.

The schedule consists of five scales, as follows: Self-care includes 10 items: poor cleanliness of clothes, poorly groomed, offensive smell, fails to wash, neglect of physical problems, unsociable habits, poor diet, incapable of budgeting, incapable of food preparation, incapable of work; Non-turbulence consists of 12 items: irresponsible behaviour, offensive behaviour, violence to others, in trouble with police, reckless behaviour, abuse of alcohol/drugs, intrusive towards others, problems with other household members, angry to others, destroys property, takes offence readily, violent to self; Social contact, six items include: withdraws from social contact, no definite interests, generally inactive, no social organization involvement, no friendships, no warmth to others; Communication, six items include: speech disordered, odd ideas in talk, intrusive in conversation, bizarre or inappropriate gestures, difficulty with conversation, reduced eye contact;

Responsibility, consists of five items: poor compliance with medication, un-cooperative with health workers, unreliable with own medication, takes others' possessions, and lacks personal property.

Each item is scored on a four point scale (1 to 4), with a score of "4" representing no problem, while a score of "1" indicates significant dysfunction. The items for each of the five scales are summed to provide a total score for that scale; a low score indicating severe disability, while a high score represents least impairment. Maximum scores are as follows: 40 for "Self-care", 48 for "Non-turbulence", 24 for "Social Contact", 24 for "Communication", and 20 for "Responsibility". A total score consists of the sum of all the items (maximum 156).

Reliability and validity
The 39 items derive from a large number of specific behaviours which were refined during pilot studies. Specific behaviours were initially selected to reduce the likelihood of global judgements (e.g. "never bathes", "never changes clothes" rather than a general dimension of "difficulty with hygiene and dress"). Items with low inter-rater reliability were removed, such as items assessing thinking and memory. Work items were deleted as few subjects were employed. The scale was further refined by principal components analysis (see Rosen *et al.*, 1989, for details). The 39 items so derived were divided into the above scales.

The total scores for each of the five scales were moderately associated with one another. A high internal consistency was reported for each scale. Inter-rater agreement was moderately high, with a mean correlation co-efficient of 0.68. Some aspects of validity were discussed by the authors, though no formal validation data were available at that time.

Utility
The schedule has been developed specifically to assist in the assessment of patients moving from hospital to the community. Though it has been used in a number of settings, experience with the scale is limited as it has only recently been developed.Unlike the other scales described, it may be administered without the need for an interview by trained staff. Its sensitivity to change has not been ascertained, and will require further investigations. The LSP incorporates measures of behavioural disturbance, but there are also a number of items which are better considered as role performance. However, because it has been gradually refined, as described above, it may be well suited to a wide variety of community settings, allowing a wide range of social disabilities to be assessed. It also provides an assessment of the degree to which behaviours are tolerated. For instance, the authors report that the most difficult behaviours for raters to accept were the patient having an offensive smell, violence, and failing to wash without reminder (Rosen *et al.*, 1989). The inter-rater agreement is reasonable, but would be expected to be better with some training.

Comparative Utility of Procedures for Assessing Social Behaviour

Before including a schedule which assesses social behaviour in any research study or other investigation a number of questions need to be asked. What are the aims of the study and why is the assessment of social behaviour of value? Which patient group is being assessed and how many patients will be included? Is social behaviour rather than other aspects of social functioning the most appropriate measure for this population? How many investigators will be available to carry out the assessments? What professional background and experience do the investigators have? Will training be necessary and available for a particular assessment instrument? How much time is available for completion of the study? How will the behavioural and other measures be analyzed? When these questions have been answered, the choice of the most appropriate instrument for assessing social behaviour in psychotic patients will be simplified.

Most of the instruments described are acceptable in terms of validity and reliability, but they differ in a number of ways, such as specific items covered, sensitivity, time of administration, and time interval covered. These differences considered together with the requirements of a particular investigation will allow the selection of the most appropriate instrument from those discussed. If patients with widely differing illness severity are being assessed, it may be necessary to combine a behavioural scale with a social role performance schedule; for example, the SBS and its complementary social role performance schedule. Alternatively, a scale such as the SBAS or the LSP may be useful. If it is required to measure the impact of impaired social functioning on a significant other, then an instrument, such as the SBAS might be considered.

If the time to complete a study is limited, those schedules which can be completed in a shorter time should be selected. For instance, in the Camden surveys (Campbell et al., 1990), the SBS proved a useful and informative instrument given the number of patients involved in the studies (over 1000) and the limited number of investigators. Other considerations in such a study are the need to maximize the co-operation of informants, and the amount of time health care professionals may have available to assist in questionnaire completion.

The interval of time covered by the instrument measuring social behaviour should be compatible with that covered by the instrument measuring psychiatric symptomatology. The Ward Behaviour Scale complements the Manchester Scale (Krawiecka et al., 1977), both of which cover a 1 week period; the SBS and the SBAS complement the PSE, covering a 1 month period. However, if a behavioural scale covering 1 month is used together with a scale assessing mental state over the preceding week, the behavioural schedule should be completed after the mental state assessment, so as to cover the period of time included in the latter.

The sensitivity of an instrument will also influence its suitability for studies which assess change as a result of treatment or other intervention. Subtle changes in social behaviour are more likely to be detected by the SBS than the WBS or

SBAS. The CBS and LSP were designed to cover a 6 month period and may be more suitable for studies covering longer periods of time.

All of the behavioural instruments discussed are relatively simple to analyze and a variety of techniques for data handling have been described for each of them. This is readily achieved by use of a microcomputer with a statistical package for the social sciences, such as SPSS or minitab (see West, 1991). This is facilitated by the scoring systems of these schedules which allow for easy data entry to the computer.

Conclusions

The instruments used to assess social behaviour in patients with psychosis were developed because of a need to measure disturbances which are seen in often very disabled patients whose abilities in the realm of role performance are also severely impaired. These two aspects of social functioning often overlap and careful consideration needs to be given to a decision which excludes one or the other. The appropriate choice of instrument requires careful planning and understanding of the aims of a study.

The assessment of social behaviour usually relies heavily on information obtained from interviewing a key informant, such as mental health worker, relative or friend. Arranging interviews with patients and relatives can be problematic and much time and energy may have to be spent repeatedly visiting homes before an assessment may be completed. The peripatetic researcher requires stamina and perseverance. The difficulty gaining access to interview patients or relatives with psychosis needs to be considered. One of us (CP) found that the assessments in the community were facilitated by first approaching mental health workers who knew the patients and families well (Pantelis *et al.*, 1988). In this way those who were familiar with the patients and their relatives could explain what was required and introduce the investigators. On the other hand relatives and friends may find the interview informative and helpful.

References

Andreasen, N. (1982). Negative symptoms in schizophrenia. *Archives of General Psychiatry,* **39**, 784-788.

Asberg, M., Montgomery, S.A., Perris, C., Schalling, D. and Sedvall, G. (1978). The comprehensive psychopathological rating scale. *Acta Psychiatrica Scandinavica,* Suppl. 271: 5-27.

American Psychiatric Association. (1987). "Diagnostic and Statistical Manual of Mental Disorders". 3rd Edn. (Revised), Washington DC.

Barnes, T.R.E., Milavic, G., Curson, D.A. and Platt, S.D. (1983). The use of the social behaviour assessment schedule (SBAS) in a trial of maintenance antipsychotic therapy in schizophrenic outpatients: pimozide versus fluphenazine. *Social Psychiatry,* **18**, 193-199.

Brewin, C.R., Wing, J.K., Mangan , S., Brugha, T.S. and MacCarthy, B. (1987). Principle and practice of measuring needs in the long term mentally ill. The MRC needs for care assessment. *Psychological Medicine,* **17**, 971-981.

Brewin, C.R., Veltro, F., Wing, J.K., MacCarthy, B. and Brugha, T.S. (1990). The assessment of psychiatric disability in the community: A comparison of clinical, staff, and family interviews. *British Journal of Psychiatry,* **157**, 671-674.

Brugha, T.S. (1989). Social psychiatry. *In* "The Instruments of Psychiatric Research", (Ed. C. Thompson), pp. 253-270, John Wiley and Sons Ltd., London.

Campbell, P.G., Taylor, J., Pantelis, C. and Harvey, C. (1990). Studies of schizophrenia in a large mental hospital proposed for closure and in two halves of an inner London borough served by the hospital. *In* "International Perspectives in Schizophrenia Research: Biological, Social and Epidemiological Findings". (Ed. M. Weller), pp. 185-202, John Libbey, London.

Curson, D.A., Barnes, T.R.E., Bamber, R.W., Platt, S.D., Hirsch, S.R. and Duffy, J.C. (1985). Long-term maintenance of chronic schizophrenic outpatients: the seven year follow-up of the MRC fluphenazine/placebo trial. III Relapse postponement or relapse prevention? The implications for longterm outcome. *British Journal of Psychiatry,* **146**, 474-480.

Curson, D.A., Pantelis, C., Ward, J. and Barnes, T.R.E. (1992). Institutionalism and schizophrenia thirty years on: Clinical poverty and the social environment in three British Mental Hospitals in 1960 compared with a fourth in 1990. *British Journal of Psychiatry,* **160**, 230-241.

Ellsworth, R. B., Foster, L., Childers, B., Arthur, G. and Kroeker, D. (1968). Hospital and community adjustment as perceived by psychiatric patients, their families and staff. *Journal of Consulting and Clinical Psychology,* **32** (No 5 Pt 2), 1-41.

Endicott, J. and Spitzer, R.L. (1972a). What! Another rating scale? The Psychiatric Evaluation Form. *Journal of Nervous and Mental Disease,* **154**, 88-104.

Endicott, J. and Spitzer, R.L. (1972b). Current and Past Psychopathology Scales (CAPPS): Rationale, reliability, and validity. *Archives of General Psychiatry,* **27**, 678-687.

Endicott, J., Spitzer, R.L., Fleiss, J. and Cohen, J. (1976). The Global Assessment Scale – A procedure for measuring overall severity of psychiatric disturbance. *Archives of General Psychiatry,* **33**, 766-771.

Gibbons, J.S., Horn, S.H., Powell, J.M. and Gibbons, J.L. (1984). Schizophrenic patients and their families: a survey in a psychiatric service based on a DGH unit. *British Journal of Psychiatry,* **144**, 70-77.

Gubman, G.D., Tessler, R.C. and Willis, G. (1987). Living with the mentally ill: factors affecting household complaints. *Schizophrenia Bulletin,* **13**(4), 727-736.

Hewett, S., Ryan, P. and Wing, J.K. (1975). Living without mental hospitals. *Journal of Social Policy,* **4**, 391-404.

Hirsch, S.R., Platt, S.D., Knights, A. and Weyman, A. (1979). Shortening hospital stay for psychiatric care: effect on patients and their families. *British Medical Journal,* **1**, 442-446.

Honigfeld, G., Gillis, R.D. and Klett, C.J. (1966). NOSIE-30, a treatment sensitive ward behaviour scale. *Psychological Reports,* **19**, 180-182.

Jaspers, K. (1963). "General Psychopathology". (Trans. from the German 7th edition, by J. Hoenig and M.W. Hamilton), Manchester University Press, Manchester.

Johnstone, E.C., Owens, D.G.C., Gold, A., Crow, T.J. and Macmillan, J.F. (1981). Institutionalisation and the defects of schizophrenia. *British Journal of Psychiatry,* **139**, 195-203.

Johnstone, E.C., Owens, D.G.C., Gold, A., Crow, T.J. and Macmillan, J.F. (1984). Schizophrenic patients discharged from hospital – A follow-up study. *British Journal of*

Psychiatry, **145**, 586-590.

Johnstone, E.C., Owens, D.G.C., Frith, C.D. and Calvert, L.M. (1985). Institutionalisation and the outcome of functional psychoses. *British Journal of Psychiatry,* **146**, 36-44.

Katz, M.M. and Lyerly, S.B. (1963). Methods for measuring adjustment and social behaviour in the community. I. Rationale, description, discriminative validity and scale development. *Psychological Reports,* **13** (Monograph suppl. 4), 503-535.

Krawiecka, M., Goldberg, D. and Vaughan, M. (1977). A standardised psychiatric assessment scale for rating chronic psychotic patients. *Acta Psychiatrica Scandinavica,* **55**, 299-308.

Liddle, P.F. (1987). The symptoms of chronic schizophrenia: a re-examination of the positive-negative dichotomy. *British Journal of Psychiatry,* **151**, 145-151.

Lorr, M. and Klett, C.J. (1967). "Inpatient Multidimensional Psychiatric Scale (IMPS) revised Manual". Consulting Psychologists Press, Palo Alto, California.

Lutz, M., Appelt, H. and Cohen, R. (1980). Belastungsfaktoren in dem Familien alkoholkranker und depresiver Frauen aus der sicht der Ehemanner. *Social Psychiatry,* **15**, 137-144.

MacCarthy, B., Liddle, P.F., Sinclair, J., Rooney, B., Kelly, J. and Warren, A. (1991). Everyday behaviour and cognitive function, (MS in submission).

Mann, S.A. and Cree, W. (1976). "New" long-stay psychiatric patients: a national survey of fifteen mental hospitals in England and Wales 1972/3. *Psychological Medicine,* **6**, 603-610.

Mann, S.A. and Sproule, J. (1972). Reasons for a six month stay. *In* "Evaluating a Community Psychiatric Service: The Camberwell Register 1964-71". (Eds J.K. Wing and A.M. Hailey), pp. 233-248. Oxford University Press, London.

McCreadie, R.G. (1982). The Nithsdale schizophrenia survey I: Psychiatric and social handicaps. *British Journal of Psychiatry,* **140**, 582-586.

McCreadie, R.G. (1990). The Nithsdale schizophrenia surveys 1981-1988: An overview. *In* "International Perspectives in Schizophrenia Research: Biological, Social and Epidemiological Findings". (Ed. M. Weller), pp. 179-183, John Libbey, London.

Overall, J.E. and Gorham, D.R. (1962). The brief psychiatric rating scale. *Psychological Reports,* **10**, 799-812.

Owens, D.G.C. and Johnstone, E.C. (1980) . The disabilities of chronic schizophrenia: their nature and the factors contributing to their development. *British Journal of Psychiatry,* **136**, 384-395.

Pantelis, C., Taylor, J. and Campbell, P.G. (1988). The South Camden Schizophrenia Survey – An experience of community based research. *Bulletin of the Royal College of Psychiatrists,* **12**(3): 98-101.

Pantelis, C., Harvey, C., Taylor, J., Campbell, P.G. (1991). The Camden Schizophrenia Surveys: symptoms and syndromes in schizophrenia (Abstract). *Biological Psychiatry,* **29**, 646S.

Platt, S. (1985). Measuring the burden of psychiatric illness on the family: an evaluation of some rating scales. *Psychological Medicine,* **15**, 383-393.

Platt, S. (1986). Evaluating social functioning. A critical review of scales and their underlying concepts. *In* "The Psychopharmacology of Schizophrenia". (Eds P.B. Bradley and S.R. Hirsch), pp. 263-285, Oxford University Press, London.

Platt, S., Weyman, A. and Hirsch, S.R. (1978). "Social Behaviour Assessment Schedule (SBAS)". 2nd Edn revised, Dept of Psychiatry, Charing Cross Hospital, London.

Platt, S., Weyman, A., Hirsch, S.R. and Hewett, S. (1980). The social behaviour assessment schedule (SBAS): rationale, contents, scoring and reliability. *Social Psychiatry,* **15,** 43-55.

Platt, S., Hirsch, S.R. and Knights, A.C. (1981). Effects of brief hospitalisation on psychiatric patients' behaviour and social functioning. *Acta Psychiatrica Scandinavica,* **63,** 117-128.

Platt, S., Weyman, A., Hirsch, S.R. and Hewett, S. (1983). "Social Behaviour Assessment Schedule (SBAS)". 3rd Edn, NFER-Nelson, Windsor.

Prusoff, B.A. Klerman, G.L. and Paykel, E.S. (1972). Pitfalls in the self-report assessment of depression. *Canadian Psychiatric Association Journal,* **17,** 101-107.

Remington, M. and Tyrer, P. (1979). The social functioning schedule – a brief semi-structured interview. *Social Psychiatry,* **14,** 151-157.

Rosen, A., Hadzi-Pavlovic, D. and Parker, G. (1989). The Life Skills Profile: A measure assessing function and disability in schizophrenia. *Schizophrenia Bulletin,* **15,** 325-337.

Ryan, P. and Wing, J.K. (1979). Residential care for the mentally disabled. *In* "Community Care for the Mentally Disabled". (Ed. J.K. Wing and R. Olsen), pp. 60-89, Oxford University Press, London.

Schubart, C., Krumm, B., Biehl, M. and Schwartz, R. (1986). Measurement of social disability in a schizophrenic patient group: Definition, assessment and outcome over two years in a cohort of schizophrenic patients of recent onset. *Social Psychiatry,* **21,** 1-9.

Spitzer, R.L. and Endicott, J.E. (1973). The value of the interview for the evaluation of psychopathology. *In* "Psychopathology: Contributions in the Biological, Behavioural and Social Sciences". (Eds J. Hammer., K. Salzinger and S. Sutton), pp. 397-408, Wiley, New York.

Spitzer, R.L., Endicott, J., Fleiss, J.L. and Cohen, J. (1970). Psychiatric Status Schedule: a technique for evaluating psychopathology and impairment of role functioning. *Archives of General Psychiatry,* **23,** 41-55.

Stevens, B. (1972). Dependence of schizophrenic patients on elderly relatives. *Psychological Medicine,* **2,** 17-32

Sturt, E. and Wykes, T. (1987). Assessment schedules for chronic psychiatric patients. *Psychological Medicine,* **17,** 485-493.

Wallace, C.J. (1986). Functional assessment in rehabilitation. *Schizophrenia Bulletin,* **12**(4), 604-630.

West, R. (1991). "Computing for Psychologists: Statistical Analysis using SPSS and Minitab". Harwood Academic Publishers, London.

Wing, J.K. (1961). A sample and reliable subclassification of chronic schizophrenia. *Journal of Mental Science,* **107,** 862-875.

Wing, J.K. (1980). Innovations in social psychiatry. *Psychological Medicine,* **10,** 219-230.

Wing, J.K. (1989). The measurement of "social disablement". The MRC social behaviour and social role performance schedules. *Social Psychiatry and Psychiatric Epidemiology,* **24**(4), 173-178.

Wing, J.K. and Brown, G.W. (1970). "Institutionalism and Schizophrenia. A Comparative Study of Three Mental Hospitals". Cambridge University Press, London; (1988). World Health Organisation. Psychiatric Disability Assessment Schedule (WHO/DAS). WHO, Geneva.

Wing, J.K., Cooper, J.E. and Sartorius, N. (1974). "The Measurement and Classification of Psychiatric Symptoms". Cambridge University Press, London.

Wykes, T. (1982). A hostel ward for "new" long-stay patients: an evaluative study of "a ward in a house". *In* "Long-term Community Care: Experience in a London Borough". (Ed. J.

K. Wing). Psychological Medicine Monograph, Supplement 2, 59-97.

Wykes, T. and Sturt, E. (1986). The measurement of social behaviour in psychiatric patients: an assessment of the reliability and validity of the SBS schedule. *British Journal of Psychiatry,* **148**, 1-11.

Wykes, T., Sturt, E. and Creer, C. (1982). Practices of day and residential units in relation to the social behaviour of attenders. *In* "Long-term Community Care: Experience in a London Borough". Psychological Medicine Monograph. Supplement 2, 15-27.

11. The Assessment of Social Functioning and Dependency in Psychiatric Rehabilitation

Sheila Stayte and Robert Pugh

As the movement to close long-stay hospitals gathers momentum, the assessment of people with long-term mental health problems has become increasingly important. New community-based services developed to replace the large institutions will need to cater not only for the existing long-stay patients but also for those people who would otherwise have been admitted for long-term care. Although modern treatment approaches have gradually reduced the extent of the need for such admissions, nevertheless, there remains a sizeable proportion of the psychiatric population, and in particular of those with psychotic conditions, whose disabilities and needs are extensive and long-lasting (Prudo and Munroe Blum, 1987). If this dual task is to be achieved, information on the nature and needs of these two groups will be required by clinicians and planners for use in both the delivery of care to individuals and also the overall design and evaluation of services.

Given that in many districts the development of replacement services is dependent upon the transfer of resources from the large institutions, the focus has inevitably tended to be on long-stay patients. From being a comparatively ignored and under-resourced section of the psychiatric population, long-stay patients now bid fair to becoming the most surveyed group in the service and the hunt has been on for the perfect instrument which will yield up all the required information and which, in particular, will assess "rehabilitation potential" and predict who will be successfully discharged.

One of the difficulties with this search is that it has, perhaps, been based on an outdated and, in some ways, simplistic view of rehabilitation. There has been an underlying assumption that "rehabilitation potential" is an intrinsic attribute of the individual and that those scoring highly on putative measures of this can be assisted to return to the community, after which they will be relatively independent of the service. This approach views rehabilitation as a one-off procedure or "treatment" relevant primarily to long-term inpatients and having a clear, desired end-point. The origins of this limited interpretation of rehabilitation are understandable given the nature of the treatment developments, sociological theory and civil rights ideology which helped to form the early de-institutionalization movement. But its persistence is to be regretted given the expectations which it may arouse in those responsible for current work and service developments.

Broader and more realistic models, with important implications for assessment, have been formulated by clinicians and researchers working with long-term clients in the community as well as the long-stay (Anthony, 1978; Royal College of Psychiatrists, 1980; Watts and Bennett, 1983; Shepherd, 1984). These conceptual developments depict rehabilitation as a continuous and "recursive" process, applicable in many service settings and having particular regard to the interaction between the individual and the environment. People with long-term mental health problems are subject to both the primary disabilities of their illness (emotional, cognitive, motivational and behavioural dysfunction) and a wide range of secondary and tertiary handicaps (loss of self-esteem and confidence, social withdrawal, loss of social roles and networks, unemployment, homelessness, poverty and stigmatization). The institutionalization of the long-stay patient is but the final compounding and reinforcing factor.

The goals of rehabilitation are to enable the individual to "make the best use of his residual abilities in order to function at an optimum level in as normal a social context as possible" (Bennett, 1978). This entails both working with the client to enhance his/her coping skills and the provision of such "prosthetic environments" and social, emotional and material supports as may be necessary to maintain that optimum level. As an outcome, independence from mental health services (whether health, social services or voluntary care) is a laudable ideal but one which may be unrealistic for many, for whom a long-term commitment on the part of the combined services is more appropriate.

From this perspective, the notion of "rehabilitation potential" evaporates. The purpose of the exercise in relation to the individual, whether in hospital or the community, is to outline his/her range of service needs and to meet these through an individually designed package of therapeutic interventions, care and practical support which is then evaluated and modified on a recurrent basis. If the idea of "potential" has any usefulness, it is perhaps best thought of as being indicated by the person's response to rehabilitative programmes and environments. This can only be observed over a period of time, which for many may be prolonged and certainly, a judgement of potential cannot be made in a vacuum. The opportunities, limitations and shaping influences present in the individual's psycho-social and physical environment need to be taken into consideration in interpreting assessments of current functioning (Mariotto and Paul, 1975). Furthermore, in a district which has a wide and flexible variety of residential, day and domiciliary services, a higher proportion of long-term patients may well be considered as having the potential to leave hospital, or avoid admission, than in a district where resources outside large-scale institutional care are limited in both range and quantity.

This refinement in theory and practice places many demands on assessment instruments at the clinical level. In addition, there are now an increasing number of organizational pressures. Long-stay hospitals are to be replaced by community-based services, entailing the transfer of patients, capital and revenue out of the institutions. Service managers require information for strategic and operational planning. They need profiles of the patient populations, which can be translated into costed service requirements – residential accommodation, day hospitals and centres, staffing and support services.

The Government White Papers on the Health Service and Community Care (DHSS, 1989; DoH 1990) incorporating many of the recommendations of the Griffiths Report (DHSS, 1988), have profound implications for the organization and delivery of care. Care management systems will be central to the new structures. Although models for these systems will be (Intagliata, 1982; Clifford and Craig, 1988; Kanter, 1989; SSI/SWSG 1991; Onyett, 1992) they have in common the designation of individual personnel to be responsible for the coordination and delivery of care packages designed on the basis of the assessed needs of the individual client. Budgetary control is recommended in order to generate flexibility, creativity and accountability in designing these packages.

At a higher organizational level, the introduction of the distinction between purchasers and providers, the use of service contracts, and the dependence of community care funding upon evidence of detailed service planning, all require the collection of data on clients, and the aggregation and translation of this into patterns of local service needs which can be costed, supplied and monitored.

Within this clinical and organizational framework, assessment information therefore may be needed for many purposes:

1   For selection of patients for specific resettlement schemes.

2   To highlight for clinical staff a person's strengths and deficits enabling them to draw up and evaluate short-term individual care-plans.

3   To inform long-term care-planning for the individual, i.e. appropriate placement and service needs in the community.

4   To be grouped with information on others in the same residence to facilitate programme design.

5   To be used by case-managers and teams in the community to design, cost, deliver and evaluate care-packages for individuals.

6   To be aggregated with information on other patients in a given population to provide data for broad service planning.

7   To specify service packages as the basis of contracts between purchasing and providing agencies.

8   For service evaluation.

9   For clinical research.

In terms of content there may be a degree of overlap between these areas but the focus and detail will vary according to the purpose. At the clinical level, where assessment information forms the basis of decisions and actions in relation to an individual, there will be, of necessity, both breadth of information and considerable detail, embracing all those aspects of a person's life which may materially affect his/her viability as an "ordinary" member of the community. Planners, on the other hand will seek a different level of data which will enable them to ascertain the requirements of broader categories of patients, although ultimately the design of a service should arise from a judicious blend of information from these two levels, together with epidemiological data and knowledge of specific, local, cultural needs and demographic trends (McAusland *et al.*, 1986; Kingsley and Towell, 1988; Shepherd, 1988). Researchers investigating a particular treatment will of course require measures specifically targeted at the relevant dependent variable, but use of a broader framework, to include other aspects of the patients' lives or functioning, may provide additional information on unpredicted sequelae of the intervention (Anthony and Farkas, 1982).

In addition to the suitability of any given instrument for the purpose intended, a number of technical and operational criteria should be met. In two seminal articles, Hall critically reviewed assessment procedures used for long-stay patients, examining 225 articles published over a 30 year period (Hall, 1979), and in more detail, 29 ward-rating scales (Hall, 1980). The majority of studies were found wanting, leading to the conclusion that "the level of awareness of general principles of assessment design and practice is not high". Hall listed the minimal criteria for acceptability of a rating scale: selection of content on a rational basis, with elimination of items having little discriminative value or low reliability or validity; specification of the observation period; availability of norms for a clearly defined group of patients; and basic reliability and validity data. Also criticized was the practice of modifying a scale, or combining items from more than one scale, without evaluation of the technical properties of the resulting instrument. Test users are also reminded that reliability is not an inherent feature of a scale but a function of the way in which it is used. Whilst careful test construction can reduce the likelihood of low reliability, in any given study the reliability of the ratings should be re-investigated and reported.

Other considerations may influence the choice. In some circumstances, the instrument will need to be sensitive to small changes over time, in others, robustness and stability of scores over moderate periods of time may be required. Wording and definitions should be easy to understand and unambiguous, particularly where a wide range of informants are to complete rating scales, and training methods for raters should be specified. The information derived should be in a format which is relevant to, and easily used by, the clinicians or planners concerned. And finally resource implications may need to be considered, in terms of manpower, time and the cost of instruments and associated software.

Given the foregoing, one may be forgiven for concluding that the search for the perfect instrument is in vain. However, there are signs that this has at least been replaced by a more realistic goal. Along with the refinement of the concept of rehabilitation, there has been a growing acceptance of the fact that there is no one perfect assessment instrument, and that it may be both appropriate and necessary to use more than one procedure (Snaith, 1981; Anthony and Farkas, 1982; Baker and Hall, 1988). Examination of articles in recent years would appear to indicate that the criticism of previous publications has been noted (Wykes and Sturt, 1986;

Wallace, 1986; Clifford *et al.*, in press). There remain a variety of instruments, but several of these now have greater clarity concerning function and a sounder research basis in their development.

The instruments discussed below are selected from those developed in the UK. The deinstitutionalization movement in America has also produced an expansion in the number of studies of rehabilitation and community care, accompanied by the development of numerous assessment tools. Wallace (1986) and Rosen *et al.* (1989) review 26 of the available assessment procedures, with details of content, format, psychometric characteristics, uses and limitations. Anthony and Farkas (1982) summarize a further 61 instruments including outcome measures for specific, focussed treatment interventions.

The Assessment Procedures

Rehabilitation Evaluation of Hall and Baker (REHAB)
(Baker and Hall, 1983)

REHAB is a rating scale specifically designed for use with long-stay patients. It was developed during the course of a 7-year research study and has been extensively investigated (Baker and Hall, 1983, 1988). The expressed intentions of the authors are that it should measure "general disability" for overall ranking or grading of patients; be usable in a wide range of settings, identify patients with the potential for living in the community; identify general targets for treatment; be sensitive to change; and be usable over a period of time by different raters to evaluate interventions.

On the basis of behaviour over 1 week raters complete 23 items in total. Seven 3-point response scales indicate frequency of occurrence of difficult or embarrassing behaviours producing a Deviant Behaviour Score (DB). Aspects of "social and everyday" behaviour are rated in 16 items each using a continuous, visual analogue response format. These 16 scores are summed to yield a General Behaviour Score (GB), which categorizes patients as "discharge potential", "moderate handicap" or "severe handicap", and also five scale scores, (social activity, speech disturbance, speech skills, self-care and community skills).

The test pack includes individual and ward profile sheets, a raters' booklet with guidelines for each item and a user's handbook. This gives the procedure for training raters, information on the development and psychometric characteristics of the scale, guidance on interpretation of findings and tables of norms for a range of patient groups.

Reliability and validity
In terms of criteria for scale construction, the careful development of REHAB is impressive. The content was selected on the basis of empirical criteria using source studies. Pilot investigations on over 800 long-term patients in a variety of settings were used to refine the scale and examine its properties. Inter-rater reliability on the

items ranged form 0.61 to 0.92. The structure of the sub-scales, derived from factor analysis, was replicated across several patient groups. Discriminant function analyses indicated that the sub-scale and GB scores differentiated patients in contrasting settings, with correct classifications ranging from 67% to 77% of the patients. Sensitivity to change has also been demonstrated (see Baker and Hall, 1988 for details of scale development and later studies).

Utility
REHAB is technically excellent. Provided raters are properly trained, good reliability levels should be achieved, and the scale is brief and easy to complete and score. It provides sound descriptive data on the social functioning of long-term patients and has been used for a variety of research, clinical and planning purposes. Its focus is clearly long-stay patient populations, though raters in day units are guided to amend the wording, which refers largely to the hospital context, and an adapted version has been used with relatives of patients in the community (Hewitt, 1983). It highlights broad areas for intervention, though more detailed investigation is necessary to design targeted care-plans for specific patients, and it does not, nor does it claim to, provide the breadth and detail necessary to formulate individualized community care packages based on a "needs profile".

In surveying populations for planning purposes, it provides useful information on the numbers in the three broad dependency categories. However, caution should perhaps be exercised in this area, particularly in relation to selection for discharge and decisions regarding individuals. The criterion group against which the cut-off point for discharge potential scores was validated were "largely psychotic day hospital attenders surviving in the community" with no information on accommodation or support services, and there are, as yet, no large-scale longitudinal studies of the relationship between REHAB scores, resettlement outcome and service profiles. In one of the DHSS Care in the Community pilot projects, of 50 people discharged for whom baseline (pre-rehabilitation) REHAB scores were available, 27 were "discharge potential", 17 were "moderate handicap" and six were "severe handicap". Readmissions included two from each category (Pugh and Stayte, in preparation). Whilst the distribution of scores broadly supports the distinction between categories, the successful discharge of those not identified as "discharge potential" argues against premature categorization of individuals as opposed to broad estimates of numbers for planning. The need for further refinements in light of the changing service context has been acknowledged by the authors and a "Mark 2" version has been proposed (Carson *et al.*, 1989).

Community Placement Questionnaire (CPQ)
(Clifford et al., 1990)

This is a recently developed instrument which aims specifically to provide planning information on the community service needs of long-stay patients. The 43-item questionnaire is designed to be used for whole hospital surveys excluding acute and dementia patients. The authors' aims were to provide a "quick, efficient and reliable method of assessing the needs of a population for planning purposes", particularly in the context of hospital rundown or closure. The CPQ covers basic demographic information, levels of social, psychiatric and physical disability, behavioural problems and future needs for accommodation and day care. The majority of the items are completed by nursing staff, on the basis of the patient's behaviour in the previous month, and using 4- or 6-point rating scales with clear descriptions of each level. Ten items cover self-care, daily living and social skills; nine concern occupation/activities, physical disability, medication compliance and social network. The presence and severity of 14 socially unacceptable behaviours and 10 forms of psychological impairment are rated according to the degree to which they might jeopardize the person's community placement and three further items give information on dangerous or criminal behaviour. Several items are completed by the "multi-disciplinary team." These require opinions to be expressed regarding the community accommodation and day care considered suitable for the patient, selecting from nine options for the former and six for the latter. All options are clearly defined.

The mean score from the 10 social functioning items is taken as an overall index of the patient's level of social functioning and the mean scores can be divided into five bands from "very poor" to "high". A "Hard to Place" score is derived from 12 weighted items. For planning purposes, accommodation types can be collapsed into three: "independent", "low dependency" and "high dependency".

Reliability and validity

This instrument also has been subject to a lengthy development process. Selection of the variables was based on a literature review and discussion with managers and clinical staff and pilot studies used to refine the content. Reliability and validity were examined in several studies. For both inter-rater and test-retest reliability the majority of Kappa coefficients of agreement were significant. Percentage agreement was calculated in two ways: for the whole scale and also a simplified analysis using a bifurcation of each item to indicate presence or absence of a problem and reduction of the nine accommodation categories to the three dependency bands. Inter-informant agreement using the latter was higher (71%-100% as against 32%-100%). The authors conclude that robust global measures can be derived from less robust individual items. Of the major variables relating to service planning, the least reliable item is the day care recommendation, with percentage agreements of 56% and 42%. This unreliability remained despite the piloting of a number of variations and it is suggested that there is an intrinsic difficulty in making judgements in this area.

The scale discriminated in the expected directions between groups of patients in a variety of wards and the patterns of disability and dependence as assessed on the CPQ conformed with the team recommendations for community placements. Correlational validity, based on the allocation of patients to accommodation categories by independent clinicians, was high. Comparison of 67 inpatients and 52 day centre attenders produced a more complex pattern, indicating that "poor social functioning alone or severe behavioural problems alone are insufficient to indicate long-term hospitalization and severity of psychological impairment did not in itself discriminate between the two groups". No comparison is reported of the Hard to Place measures, which one might suppose would be affected by this pattern and which is germane to the purpose of the scale. A lack of clear discrimination on this score between the groups, however, would not necessarily invalidate the concept of hard to place clients since community presence and survival of disturbed and dependent patients may result from a variety of factors.

Utility
For the potential user, norms are available from surveys carried out in five hospitals (Clifford *et al.,* 1990). The data can be analyzed using a computer package and RDP offer survey services ranging from training and advising local personnel to carrying out a full hospital survey, analysis of the data and production of a comprehensive report. The CPQ is the first instrument specifically designed to be used as a service planning tool with long-term patients and as such is a valuable contribution. Complementary scales and questionnaires addressing individual care-planning, clients' views and community services utilization are also being developed by RDP, providing a battery of purpose-specific instruments.

Social Performance Schedules (SPS)
(MRC Social Psychiatry Unit)

Two scales for use with long-term patients have been developed by the MRC Social Psychiatry Unit at the Institute of Psychiatry, London. They are measures of social functioning, which have been designed to detect small changes in behaviour to allow evaluation of a service or treatment regime. A number of versions have been developed over the years and the Social Behaviour Schedule (SBS) and Social Role Performance Schedule (SRP) are now known jointly as the Social Role Performance Schedules (SPS) (Wykes and Sturt, 1986) (see also Chapter 10). Both schedules are completed by a trained assessor following interview with a key member of the care staff, usually a charge nurse or day centre or hostel supervisor. It is recommended that the informant is someone with a high degree of contact with the patient.

The SBS is concerned with specific behavioural problems. Twenty-one items are rated on 4 or 5 point scales. Eight describe aspects of interpersonal social behaviour; five are symptom-related; and eight cover activity level, self-care, destructiveness and mannerisms with one item for "other behaviours which impede progress". Symptoms are only rated if they result in behavioural disturbance. Anchoring descriptions and detailed instructions provide guidelines for the ratings. The data have normally been reported as the percentage of people in the target group rated at 2-4 on each item, though in a recent study (Wykes and Sturt, *op. cit.*) the calculation of a "severe problems score" and a "severe and mild problems score" is described. The measure originates in the work of Wing (1961) and Wing and Brown (1970) with long-term inpatients and was further developed in studies of the new long-stay (Mann and Cree, 1976) hostel populations (Hewett *et al.,* 1975) and long-term patients in the community (Wykes *et al.,* 1982). Reasonable levels of inter-rater and inter-informant reliability and evidence of discriminative validity are reported in Wykes and Sturt (1986).

The SRP aims to measure performance in eight commonly accepted social functions or roles: household management (HM), employment (EM), management of money (MM), child care (CC), intimate relationships (IR), other relationships (OR), presentation of self (SP), and coping with emergencies (CE). Information may be supplemented by interview with the patients themselves. Ratings in each area produce eight "disablement scores" and a "total disablement" score is derived from the percentage of role areas in which the client is totally disabled. Unlike many clinical scales, norms are available for the general population as well as groups of psychiatric patients. The schedule has been used in a number of studies (Leff and Vaughn, 1971; Wing *et al,* 1971; Stevens, 1972; Sturt and Wykes, 1987) providing data on long-term patients in both hospital and community settings.

Utility

Sturt and Wykes (1987) investigated the relationship between the SBS, the SRP and the Present State Examination (Wing *et al.,* 1974). Scores on SBS and SRP were correlated but neither showed any relationship with the PSE. Detailed examination of the data indicated that although the SRP differentiated between groups of patients in contrasting settings, the SRP score could not be used to determine the placement of patients because of the degree of overlap. The authors suggest that the SBS may be more suitable for describing the functioning of long-term hospital and hospital-hostel residents, as it covers the more severe range of disability, whilst the SRP may be more suitable for use with patients in day care only or in active rehabilitation programmes.

Morningside Rehabilitation Status Scale (MRSS)
(Affleck and McGuire, 1984)

Unlike the majority of assessment scales, the MRSS uses a small number of global ratings of broad areas of functioning, rather than a detailed, multi-item format. The authors suggest that the instrument be used as an outcome measure "at each stage of rehabilitation", so that "progress ... is accurately charted" (Affleck and McGuire, 1984; McCreadie *et al.,* 1987). Applicability to all settings and ease of use are additional aims.

The scale is completed by "a professional", on the basis of discussion with the patient and, if necessary, with staff or relatives and with the use of an *aide-memoire* check list of aspects to be covered. Four areas of functioning are each rated 0-7, with high scores representing poor performance and five of the points anchored by description. The Dependency Scale is a judgement of the extent to which the person relies on others (as indicated by living setting, staff contact, carer support, etc.); the Inactivity Scale relates to involvement, initiative and sustained interest in productive activity, both employment and leisure; a Social Integration/Isolation Scale covers the individual's ability to participate in and maintain relationships; and the Effects of Current Symptoms and Deviant Behaviour Scale portrays the extent to which impairment limits the person's way of life and affects others. Four scale scores and a total score are produced. The latter may be used to indicate high, moderate or low-level functioning.

Reliability and validity

The content was selected on the basis of previous outcome studies, with two of the scales being adaptations of measures described in the WHO (1980) discussion document – An International Classification of Impairments, Disabilities and Handicaps. Retrospective, repeated application of the measures to groups of patients undergoing rehabilitation ($n = 161$) and later comparison studies of patients in different settings ($n = 147$) were used to refine and tighten the definitions. Inter-rater reliability figures in two studies (all ratings by psychiatrists) were good, though the agreement between raters on the absolute level of performance on the Inactivity Scale remained low despite refinements. Outcome measures of patients undergoing rehabilitation showed small but significant changes in average total score and the scores of patients in various settings (outpatient clinic, two types of day care and long-stay ward) differed in the expected direction. A study of the relationship between scale scores and the presence/absence of specific problems is cited as indicating that the four scales tap different aspects. However, scores on the scales are correlated and factor analysis indicated that 72% of the variance could be accounted for by one factor. In a comparison with other assessment instruments (McCreadie *et al.*, 1987) MRSS total score correlated significantly with both the Manchester Scale (see Chapter 2 for description) which rates symptoms only, and the SAS-SR (Social Adjustment Scale by Self-Report). The scale has also been used in a study of new long-term patients (McCreadie *et al.*, 1983).

Utility

Given the restricted number of items and the global nature of the ratings, with each scale covering several features of the dimension in question, more extensive investigation of the properties and power of the instrument would perhaps be helpful. In comparison with other instruments its usefulness *per se* for either detailed individual care-planning or service design might be questioned. It reflects best perhaps, as its title indicates, the clinical team's broad summary of the person's status. It does, however, meet the criteria of speed and ease of use. The authors suggest that a clinician who knows the patient well could carry out the ratings in a few minutes and that its use may be integrated into day-to-day practice, for example by completing the scale at the end of a case review.

Functional Performance Record (FPR)
(Mulhall, 1986)

The FPR, first described by Mulhall (1986) provides a highly detailed analysis of the "actions, behaviour and functioning of those ... [with] ... physical or mental or psychiatric disabilities for use in goal-setting, evaluating outcomes, monitoring standards of care, service planning and research". It is designed to be used with any client group whose independence is impaired, irrespective of diagnosis or aetiology and concentrates exclusively on functional capacity.

The FPR contains 777 items grouped in 27 areas of functioning or "topics"; (areas considered to be irrelevant to an individual may be omitted). The 27 topics include aspects of sensory, physical and cognitive impairment, social behaviour and daily living and survival skills. Each item within a topic is rated according to clearly specified codes. A paper and pencil version can be used by care staff to identify areas for intervention, produce a baseline and evaluate care-plans. Software packages are available which generate individual bar-chart profiles of "percentage deficit" in each topic and also for the analysis and manipulation of group data. The material available includes full instructions for use of both versions plus training notes for staff on techniques for interventions in each functional area.

Utility
The author states that the major use of the FPR is "to facilitate day-to-day management of individuals" and describes it as an observational procedure as much as an assessment tool. The content selection and the task analysis format of some of the items may offer a systematic and objective delineation of behavioural functioning and a basis for the design of targeted care-plans, particularly in residential care settings.

MRC Needs for Care Assessment
(Brewin et al., 1987)

In clinical practice the easy translation of valid and relevant assessment information into individualized care packages and the subsequent monitoring of the delivery of care is essential. The MRC Needs for Care Assessment (Brewin *et al.*, 1987, 1988); Brugha *et al.*, 1988) addresses this issue in the development of a systematic procedure to specify which of a patient's problems are receiving appropriate treatment.

The first stage requires the regular and systematic assessment of functioning. Nine areas of symptoms and behavioural problems and 12 of personal and social skills are listed, and it is suggested that these may be assessed using "appropriate standardized instruments" with staff, carers and the client as informants. (In research studies, adaptations of the SBS were used). Criteria are set for the minimum acceptable levels of functioning, with guidelines on appropriate discrimination between lack of competence and lack of performance through choice.

A list of potentially effective interventions is provided for each problem area. In the second stage, each relevant intervention is rated, indicating whether it has been tried within a specified timescale and found ineffective, not yet adequately tried, currently being implemented and so on. The third stage outlines the "need status" of the client, by relating the functional assessment to the pattern of clinical work and service provision, as indicated by the intervention ratings. The result is a profile identifying those needs which are being met, those which are unmet and areas where there is no need, with recommendations for actions following on automatically from the information on interventions available but not tried. The designation of the need status in relation to any given area of functioning follows clearly defined rules. For example, there is an unmet need where the functioning is below the accepted level and it has attracted only partly effective or no intervention, and when other interventions of greater potential effectiveness exist. Over-provision of service can be identified where unnecessary interventions are being used. Where there is a significant problem, but all potential interventions have failed, the status becomes, at least on a temporary basis, "no need" with recommendations to review at a later date.

Reliability and validity
The areas of functioning, interventions and decision rules for the procedure were generated using a questionnaire survey of 50 specialist rehabilitation workers and the judgements of a research team of experienced psychiatrists and clinical psychologists. The procedure has been used in a survey of 145 long-term patients in psychiatric day care (Brugha *et al.,* 1988) and there is some evidence of reasonable reliability and validity (Brewin *et al., op. cit.*) given the ambitious nature of the procedure and the early stage of its development.

Utility
Clinical teams might question the range of areas of functioning, for example, problems with money or housing are included with symptoms and behavioural problems under the heading "distress", whereas many teams might consider it appropriate to have such service needs listed in their own right. One might also argue for some acknowledgement in the model of the way in which clinicians explore alternative hypotheses concerning the cause of a particular problem, before selecting an intervention, rather than what might be seen as simple selection from a "shopping list". Some teams also try to aim for enhancement of functioning rather than settling for the minimal acceptable level and the definition of "no need", when there is an unsuccessfully treated problem, can be difficult for staff to accept, though it has the merit of permitting the team to cease unrewarding effort at least temporarily. Despite these possible criticisms, the procedure is a major contribution to improving the quality of services to long-term clients. It incorporates an explicit model of clinical practice and increases the likelihood of comprehensive assessment of needs and systematic provision of such skilled interventions and services as are available. It also has potential for evaluating the effectiveness of a service

and could offer an appropriate framework for clinical audit in rehabilitation and community care.

The Assessment of Functioning and Need by Clients and Families

The majority of scales available draw primarily on the judgements of professional staff and service providers but the engagement of clients as active participants is now recognized as important, both in terms of the success of therapeutic programmes and the relevance of the services.

The design of measures to tap patients' motivation, preferences and perceptions of their own needs presents a number of problems, notably the suggested passivity and compliance of long-term patients, lack of knowledge of options available, poor concentration and difficulties in grasping abstract concepts. In good clinical practice with the individual, this may be addressed by taking time to get to know the person, ensuring he/she has opportunities to sample alternative settings and encouraging participation in discussion and decision-making. But the collection of valid information from groups of patients necessitates careful attention to the assessment method. Waisman and Rowland (1989) have developed an instrument to measure the relative importance that individuals attribute to various needs, using a methodology designed to be suitable for severely disabled psychiatric patients. Six statements for each of 10 areas of need associated with stress, distress and survival in the community are used in a card-sorting format to rank their relative importance. An investigation of the measure using data from long-term service users indicated good internal consistency of statements within categories, good temporal consistency and a high level of co-operation and concentration on the part of the patients.

A related study (Thapa and Rowland, 1989) looked at staff and patient perceptions of the degree to which nine areas of life contributed to overall satisfaction and happiness, using a 38-item quality-of-life questionnaire. Although there was some degree of overlap, there were also significant differences between the two groups, reinforcing the need for adequate consultation with clients, to ensure that relevant services and individual care packages are provided. The assessment of clients' and carers' views clearly merits further work, as does the related issue of the measurement of quality of life as an indicator of good rehabilitation and continuing care services.

Although few long-stay patients being resettled in the community may return to live with their families (PSSRU, 1989) the replacement of hospital care by community-based rehabilitation services makes inclusion of carers' needs and experiences highly pertinent.

Social Behaviour Assessment Schedule (SBAS)
(Platt et al., 1980, 1983) (see also Chapter 10)

The SBAS was designed to provide a comprehensive assessment of symptomatic behaviour, social role performance and objective and subjective burden on members of the household. An interview is conducted with a significant other, providing information and ratings on 329 items divided into six sections: demographic data, symptoms and resulting distress, social role performance, well-being of the household in relationships to the patient's illness, stressful life events, and support received. Six scores reflect aspects of the patient's disturbance and dependency and objective and subjective burden.

Reliability and validity

Inter-rater reliability for most of the summary scores is high, the exception being subjective distress and the authors suggest that this should be assessed at an item level rather than as a global measure. Sensitivity of the "burden" scales to changes in the patient's behaviour has been demonstrated (Platt and Hirsch, 1981). Platt (1985) reviews other measures of family burden, and the Life Skills Profile (Rosen *et al.,* 1989) also includes a "hard to take" measure of the impact of client's behaviour on relatives and care staff.

Concluding Comments

It is arguable that the distinction between assessment in rehabilitation and assessment in other aspects of psychiatry covered in this book is somewhat artificial. The formulation of an individual's pattern of therapeutic and service needs may well require the use of procedures described in other chapters. Conversely, Watts and Bennett (*op. cit.*) suggest that the rehabilitation approach has much to offer a great number of service-users and could beneficially be integrated in the general routine care of psychiatric patients.

Nevertheless, the design of assessment procedures specifically for use in services for people with long-term mental health problems remains a valid undertaking. The potential investigator should be clear as to the purpose of the particular data collection exercise and the nature of the information required, selecting the most appropriate instrument and using more than one if necessary. Training of interviewers and raters is vital, as is an awareness of the inevitable limitations of any given instrument and caution in the interpretation of the results. With these provisos, the recent developments in this field are encouraging and offer a choice of procedures which, if appropriately used, may help to improve the quality of services in rehabilitation and community care.

References

Affleck, J.W. and McGuire, R.J. (1984). The measurement of psychiatric rehabilitation status: a review of the needs and a new scale. *British Journal of Psychiatry,* **145,** 517-525.

Anthony, W.A. (1978). "The Principles of Psychiatric Rehabilitation". University Park Press, Baltimore.

Anthony, W.A. and Farkas, M. (1982). A client outcome planning model for assessing psychiatric rehabilitation interventions. *Schizophrenia Bulletin,* **8,** no 1. 13-28.

Anthony, W.A. *et al.* (1980). "Skills of Rehabilitation Programming". University Park Press. Baltimore.

Baker, R. and Hall, J.N. (1983). "Rehabilitation Evaluation of Hall and Baker (REHAB)". Vine Publishing Ltd., Aberdeen.

Baker, R. and Hall, J.N. (1988). REHAB: a new assessment instrument for chronic psychiatric patients. *Schizophrenia Bulletin,* **14**, no. 1, 97-11.

Bennett, D.H. (1978). Social forms of psychiatric treatment in schizophrenia. *In* "Towards a New Synthesis". (Ed. J.K. Wing). Academic Press, London.

Brewin, C.R., Wing, J.K., Mangen, T.S. *et al.* (1987). Principles and practice of measuring needs in the long-term mentally-ill: the M.R.C. Needs for Care Assessment. *Psychological Medicine,* **17**, 971-981.

Brewin, C.R., Wing, J.K., Mangen, T.S. *et al.* (1988). Needs for care among the long-term mentally-ill: a report from the Camberwell High Contact Survey. *Psychological Medicine,* **18**, 457-468.

Brugha, T.S., Wing, J.K., Brewin, C.R., MacCarthy, B., Mangen, S., Lesage, A. and Mumford, J. (1988). The problems of people in long-term psychiatric care: An introduction to the Camberwell High Contact Survey. *Psychological Medicine,* **18**, 443-456.

Carson, J., Croucher, P. and Abrahamson, D. (1989). "Using REHAB in Rehabilitation and Resettlement". Proceedings of a Symposium. Waltham Forest Health Authority, Mental Health Unit, Claybury Hospital.

Clifford, P. and Graig, T. (1988). "Case Management Systems for the Long-term Mentally Ill". National Unit for Psychiatric Research and Development.

Clifford, P., Charman, A., Webb, Y., Craig, T.J.K. and Cowan, D. (1990). Planning for Community Care: 1. The Community Placement Questionnaire. Submitted for publication.

Clifford, P., Charman, A., Webb, Y. and Betts, S. (1990). Planning for Community Care: 2. Long-stay Populations of Hospitals Scheduled for Rundown or Closure. Submitted for publication.

D.H.S.S. (1989). "Caring for People: Community Care in the Next Decade and Beyond". H.M.S.O. London.

D.H.S.S. (1989). "Working for Patients: Caring for the 1990s". H.M.S.O. London.

Dott. (1990). "N.H.S. and Community Care Act 1990". H.M.S.O., London.

Griffiths, R. (1988). "Community Care: Agenda for Action". H.M.S.O. London.

Hall, J.N. (1979). Assessment procedures used in studies on long-stay patients: a survey of papers published in the British Journal of Psychiatry. *British Journal of Psychiatry,* **135**, 330-335.

Hall, J.N. (1980). Ward rating scales for long-stay patients: a review. *Psychological Medicine,* **10**, 277-288.

Hewitt, K.E. (1983). The behaviour of schizophrenic day-patients at home: an assessment by relatives. *Psychological Medicine,* **13**, 885-889.

Intagliata, J. (1982). Improving the quality of life of community care for the chronically mentally disabled: the role of case management. *Schizophrenia Bulletin,* **8**, No 4

Kanter, J. (1989). Clinical case management: definition, principles, components. *Hospital and Community Psychiatry,* **40**, 361-369.

Kingsley, S. and Towell, D. (1988). Planning for high-quality local services. *In* "Community Care in Practice: Services for the the Continuing Care Client". (Eds A. Lavender and F.

Holloway). John Wiley, Chichester.

Leff, J. and Vaughn, C. (1971). Psychiatric patients in contact and out of contact with services: a clinical and social assessment. *In* "Evaluating a Community Psychiatric Service". (Eds J.K. Wing and A.M. Haley). pp.259-274. Oxford University Press, London.

McAusland, T., Towell, D. and Kingsley, S. (1986). Assessment, rehabilitation and resettlement. *In* "Psychiatric Services in Transition". Paper No. 2. King's Fund College, London.

McCreadie, R.G., Wilson, A. and Burton, L. (1983). The Scottish survey of "New Chronic" inpatients. *British Journal of Psychiatry*, **143**, 564-571.

McCreadie, R.G., Affleck, J.W., McKenzie, Y. and Robinson, O.T. (1987). A comparison of scales for assessing rehabilitation patients. *British Journal of Psychiatry*, **151**, 520-522.

Mann, S. and Cree, W. (1976). "New" long-stay psychiatric patients. A national sample of fifteen mental hospitals in England and Wales, 1972/3. *Psychological Medicine*, **6**, 603-616.

Mariotto, M.J. and Paul, G.L. (1975). Persons versus situations in the real-life functioning of chronically institutionalised mental patients. *Journal of Abnormal Psychology*, **84**, 483-493.

Mulhall, D.J. (1986). The Functional Performance Record: An observational procedure for use with disabled people. *Behavioural Psychotherapy*, **14**, 69-80.

Mulhall, D.J. (1989). "Functional Performance Record". NFER-Nelson, Windsor.

Onyett, S. (1992). "Case Management in Mental Health". Chapman and Hall, London.

Platt, S. (1985). Measuring the burden of psychiatric illness on the family: an evaluation of some rating scales. *Psychological Medicine*, **15**, 383-393.

Platt, S. and Hirsch, S. (1981). The effects of brief hospitalization upon psychiatric patient's household. *Acta Psychiatrica Scandinavica*, **64**, 199-126.

Platt, S., Weyman, A., Hirsch, S. and Hewitt, S. (1980). The social behaviour assessment schedule (SBAS). Rationale, contents, scoring and reliability of a new interview schedule. *Social Psychiatry*, **15**, 43-55.

Platt, S., Weyman, A. and Hirsch, S. (1983). "Social Behaviour Assessment Schedule (SBAS)". 3rd Edn. NFER-Nelson, Windsor, Berks.

Prudo, R. Munroe, and Blum, M. (1987). Five-year outcome and prognosis in schizophrenia: a report from the London field research centre of the international pilot study of schizophrenia. *British Journal of Psychiatry*, **150**, 345-354.

P.S.S.R.U. (1989). Care in the community: final report discussion paper 615. Personal Social Services Research Unit. University of Kent at Canterbury.

Rosen, A., Hadzi-Pavlovic, D. and Parker, G. (1989). The life skills profile: a measure assessing function and disability in schizophrenia. *Schizophrenia Bulletin*, **15**, No. 2, 325-337.

Royal College of Psychiatrists (1980). "Psychiatric Rehabilitation in the 1980s". Report of the working party on rehabilitation of the social and community psychiatry section.

Shepherd, G. (1984). "Institutional Care and Rehabilitation". Longman Group Ltd.

Shepherd, G. (1988). Evaluation and service planning. *In* "Community Care in Practice: Services for the Continuing Care Client". (Eds A. Lavender and F. Holloway). John Wiley, Chichester.

Snaith, R.P. (1981). Rating Scales. *British Journal of Psychiatry*, **138**, 512-514.

S.S.I./SWSG. (1991). "Care Management and Assessment:Summary of Practice". HMSO.

Stevens, B.C. (1972). Dependence of schizophrenic patients on elderly relatives. *Psychological Medicine*, **2**, 17-32.

Sturt, E. and Wykes, T. (1987). Assessment schedules for chronic psychiatric patients. *Psychological Medicine,* **17**, 485-493.

Thapa, K. and Rowland, L. (1989). Quality of life perspectives in long-term care: staff and patient perceptions. *Acta Psychiatrica Scandinavica,* **80**, 267-271.

Waisman, L.C. and Rowland, L.A. (1989). Ranking of needs: a new method of assessment for use with chronic psychiatric patients. *Acta Psychiatrica Scandinavica,* **80**, 260-266.

Wallace, C.J. (1986). Functional assessment in rehabilitation. *Schizophrenia Bulletin,* **12**, No. 4. 604-630.

Watts, F.N. and Bennett, D.H. (1983). The concept of rehabilitation. *In* "Theory and Practice of Psychiatric Rehabilitation". (Eds F.N. Watts and D.H. Bennett). John Wiley, Chichester.

Wing, J.K. (1961). A simple and reliable subclassification of chronic schizophrenia. *Journal of Mental Science*, **107**, 826-875.

Wing, J.K. and Brown, G.W. (1970). "Institutionalization and Schizophrenia". Cambridge University Press, Cambridge.

Wing, J.K., Cooper, J.E. and Sartorius, N. (1974). "Measurement and Classification of Psychiatric Symptoms". Cambridge University Press, Cambridge.

Wing, L., Wing, J.K., Griffiths, D. and Stevens, B. (1971). An epidemiological and experimental evaluation of industrial rehabilitation of chronic psychotic patients in the community. *In* "Evaluating a Community Psychiatric Service". (Eds J.K. Wing and A.M. Haley). pp. 283-308. Oxford University Press, London.

Wykes, T. and Sturt, E. (1986). The measurement of social behaviour in psychiatric patients: an assessment of the reliability and validity of the SBS schedule. *British Journal of Psychiatry,* **148**, 1-11.

Wykes, T., Sturt, E. and Creer, C. (1982). Practices of day and residual units in relation to the social behaviour of attenders. *In* "Long-term Community Care: experience in a London Borough". *Psychological Medicine* Monograph Supplement, 2, 15-27.

12. The Differentiation of Organic and Functional Psychoses

Shôn Lewis and Janis Flint

It has long been recognized that coarse brain disease can occasionally give rise to symptoms such as persistent delusions and hallucinations in the absence of evidence of gross cognitive impairment. A range of uncommon organic conditions can mimic schizophrenia and related psychoses and this chapter will attempt to draw guidelines about clinical and neuropsychological methods of detecting such cases. Such guidelines are not clearcut and this is to some extent inevitable given that the nosological division between organic and functional psychosis is increasingly blurred. Present-day thinking is that all psychotic illness has at some level an organic substrate. However, there are two broad categories where the distinction is more clearcut. The first category is where delusions and hallucinations stem from the cerebral involvement of a named disease which affects the central nervous system: systematic lupus erythematosus, Huntington's disease, Wilson's disease, and so on. The second class which may overlap into the first, is that where delusions and hallucinations arise in the context of a demonstrable brain lesion. This latter area has become considerably more important since the advent of computerized neuroimaging techniques in the past 15 years.

The Concept of Organic Psychosis

Schizophrenia and manic depressive psychosis are classified by the World Health Organisation (1978) as "functional" or "non-organic" psychoses. These terms are unfortunate since confusion has arisen as to the ways in which the words "organic" and "non-organic" have been used. In the past they have been used on the one hand to implicate an organic cause and on the other to describe particular classes of symptoms. In ICD9 it is explicitly the latter descriptive use which is intended. Thus an "organic" psychosis is one which occurs in the presence of organic features of the mental state, such as impairment of consciousness and gross dysfunction of cognition. In more recent classification systems, such as DSMIII, DSMIIIR and the forthcoming ICD10, the use of the term has shifted to the first meaning, implying cause. Thus, separate categories of "organic mental disorders" have been introduced. Cases of psychosis without cognitive impairment, but in the presence of "evidence from the history, physical examination, or laboratory tests of a specific organic factor judged to be aetiologically related" (DSMIII), are now called "organic delusional syndrome" or "organic hallucinosis" depending on the predominant symptoms. Nevertheless in DSMIII it is acknowledged that symptoms in these "organic" mental disorders can be "essentially identical with schizophrenia". These newer classificatory systems have been said to put the diagnostician in the problematic position of having to rename a syndrome whenever a likely organic cause becomes apparent (Lewis *et al.*, 1987). Nevertheless, this convention is increasingly accepted and it forms the way in which we define organic psychosis in this chapter: namely the occurrence of psychotic phenomena, in particular delusions and hallucinations, in the absence of any major cognitive impairment but in the presence of strong evidence of a causative organic CNS lesion or disease.

This review will concentrate particularly on schizophrenia-like disorders, since these present the greatest management problem. The literature on associations between psychotic symptoms and organic disorder is vast and it is not our intention to review this here. The textbook by Lishman (1987) remains a definitive text.

The Co-occurrence of Schizophrenia-like Symptoms and Organic Brain Disease

In 1969 Kenneth Davison and Christopher Bagley published a review of the world literature, backed with some 800 references, of the co-occurrence of schizophrenia-like symptoms and organic disease. This review remains the most important work in the field and, since it is not now widely available, their main findings and conclusions will be summarized here.

The review took as its starting point the operational criteria for schizophrenia of the 1957 WHO Committee which were adapted slightly by Davison and Bagley so that their case material included cases which today would broadly be headed under the rubric of schizophrenia and paranoid psychosis. Criteria included the absence of impaired consciousness and the absence of prominent affective symptoms. The authors concluded that the occurrence of schizophrenia-like symptoms exceeded chance expectation in many organic CNS disorders and that where a discrete lesion was present, those in the temporal lobe and diencephalon seemed to be particularly significant. They also noted that any distinguishing clinical features between organic and functional schizophrenia were "largely illusory", although we will return to this later. They noted that such organic psychoses usually occurred in patients without genetic loading for schizophrenia.

Davison and Bagley reviewed evidence for a large range of individual CNS disorders. Epilepsy was statistically associated with schizophrenia-like psychosis, particularly where a temporal lobe lesion existed. Head injury was also a risk factor for psychosis, again with a possible association with temporal lobe lesions, although severe closed head injury with diffuse cerebral damage was related to early development of psychotic symptoms. Encephalitic disorders, including cerebral syphilis, Wilson's disease, Huntington's disease, Friedreich's ataxia, vitamin B12 deficiency, subarachnoid haemorrhage, and cerebral tumour also seemed to be associated with an increased risk of schizophrenia-like symptoms.

There was much less evidence to implicate other CNS disorders such as multiple sclerosis, motor neurone disease and Parkinson's disease.

It should not be surprising that 20 years later a few of Davison's and Bagley's conclusions might be amended. For example, their finding of an association between narcolepsy and psychosis would now be explained by most authorities on the basis of the use of amphetamines in treatment, rather than the disease itself. The correlation between cerebral tumour and schizophrenia-like symptoms is probably not as strong as once thought. The problem here is that most studies looked at this correlation by retrospective autopsy studies, in which it is usually difficult to date the onset of the tumour as being before the onset of the symptoms of psychosis. Many such instances could be better explained as chance association, unless the tumours were of the type whose natural history was very long standing. Conversely, new evidence for other disorders being associated is now available. A present day list would also include sex chromosome abnormalities, Cushing's syndrome, thyroid and parathyroid disorders, cerebral sarcoidosis, SLE and, most recently, AIDS. There does seem to be a small group of people with demyelinating disorders, in particular Schilder's disease and multiple sclerosis specifically involving temporal lobe sites, which can also present with psychotic symptomatology. Recent reviews relevant to this area include those of Cummings (1985), Cutting (1987) and Johnstone et al.(1988), as well as a review of congenital disorders (Lewis, 1989).

How Common are Organic Psychoses?

The prevalence of organic psychoses within psychiatric populations is unknown. One difficulty in estimating the rate of the problem is definition: how confident can one be that an uncovered brain lesion is truly responsible for the presenting psychotic symptoms ? A second difficulty is that the closer one looks the more likely it is that organic pathology will be revealed. The widespread availability of non-invasive brain imaging techniques has shown that unsuspected cerebral lesions occur in a small but significant number of patients with schizophrenic symptoms. Most structural brain imaging research in psychosis has concentrated on minor, quantitative changes involving widened fluid spaces (Table 1).

TABLE 1. *Replicated CT Scan changes found in schizophrenia and bipolar disorder.*

1	Minor lateral ventricular enlargement.
2	Minor third ventricle enlargement.
3	Widened cortical sulci and fissures.

These minor degrees of enlargement of ventricles and sulci found in the majority of studies would not usually be reported as abnormal by most clinical radiologists. However, there are a handful of reports in the literature of gross focal brain lesions in schizophrenia. There have been case reports of schizophrenia in association with aqueduct stenosis arachnoid and septal cysts (Kuhnley *et al.,* 1981; Lewis and Mezey, 1985) as demonstrated on CT. Three larger studies enable an estimate to be made of the prevalence of such focal lesions in schizophrenia. Owens *et al.* (1980) in their series of 136 schizophrenic patients found "unsuspected intracranial pathology" as a focal finding on CT in 12 cases (9%), excluding lesions due to leucotomy. This was a relatively elderly sample: five of these 12 cases were aged over 65. In an unpublished series, Lewis (1987) examined a series of 228 Maudsley Hospital patients who met RDC for schizophrenia and who had been consecutively scanned for clinical reasons. Patients with a history of epilepsy or intracranial surgery, or who were aged over 65 at the time of scan, were excluded. The original scan reports were examined and the films of those not unequivocally normal were reappraised by a neuroradiologist blind to the original report. In 41 patients the scan showed a definite intracranial abnormality. This was in the nature of enlarged fluid spaces in 28 cases, but in 13 patients (6%) there was a discrete focal lesion. These lesions varied widely in location and probable pathology (Table 2), although left temporal and right parietal regions were most commonly implicated.

TABLE 2. *Laterality, locus and nature of focal lesions found on CT in 13 of 228 schizophrenic patients.*

Site	Number	Nature of lesion
Right-sided		
frontal	1	Low attenuation
parietal	3	Calcified mass 1
		Porencephalic cyst 1
		Low attenuation 1
temporal	1	Old abscess cavity
Left-sided		
frontoparietal	1	Low attenuation
temporal	3	Arachnoid cyst 2
occipitotemporal	1	Calcification 1
		Arachnoid cyst
Midline	1	Septal cyst
Bilateral	2	Occipital low attenuation 1
		Parasagittal calcification 1

The third study (Lewis and Reveley, in preparation) was an attempt to examine a geographically defined sample of schizophrenic patients, ascertained as part of a large multi-disciplinary survey. All Camberwell residents who, on a particular census day, were aged between 18 and 65 and were in regular contact with any psychiatric day service, were approached. Of 120 eligible people, 83 consented to CT and psychiatric interview. Fifty of these met Research Diagnositic Criteria for schizophrenia or schizoaffective disorder. In four of these 50 patients (8%), were found clinically unsuspected focal lesions: low density in the right caudate head; a left occipitotemporal porencephalic cyst; low density regions in the right parietal lobe; agenesis of the corpus callosum (see below). None of 50 matched healthy volunteers showed focal pathology on CT.

Given the differences in the nature of the patient sample, these three studies are in rough agreement about the prevalence of unexpected focal abnormalities on CT: between 6% and 9%. A similar figure emerged from the important study of Johnstone and colleagues (1988). In this study, the sample was a consecutive one of 328 patients presenting with an episode of psychosis, aged between 15 and 70 years. Patients were screened clinically, without diagnostic neuroimaging, for the presence of organic illnesses which the authors judged was "of definite or possible aetiological significance" for the psychotic symptoms. Twenty-four (7%) patients fell into the category, with the following diagnoses: amphetamine abuse (2); alcohol abuse (2); polydrug and other abuse (8), syphilis (1), thyroid disease (2); stroke (1); frontal tumour (1); pituitary tumour (1); steroid treatment (1); systemic lupus erythrematosus (1); carcinoma of lung (1); B12 avitaminosis (1); diabetes mellitus (1).

Distinguishing Organic and Functional Psychoses: Theory

Both brain imaging and clinical studies, as reviewed above, point to a prevalence rate of 5-8% for psychoses of likely organic aetiology amongst series of relatively unselected patients. If this is the case, is it possible to distinguish the minority of organic cases on clinical grounds alone?

The short answer is no, in that there is a large overlap in presenting symptoms between functional and organic psychoses. Nonetheless, several studies have compared symptom profiles in the two groups and some general differences do emerge.

In their review of the literature, Davison and Bagley (1969) compared rates of individual psychotic symptoms in 150 reported cases of various organic schizophrenia-like psychoses with a series of 475 patients with functional schizophrenia reported by other authors. Of 14 clinical features compared, six occurred significantly less frequently in the organic group: flat or incongruous affect; passivity feelings; thought disorder; auditory hallucinations; tactile hallucinations; schizoid premorbid personality; family history of schizophrenia. Catatonic symptoms were reported more frequently in organic cases. Sixty-four per cent of the organic group showed Schneiderian first rank symptoms, although this feature was not recorded in the control group. These results are intriguing, although they represent a retrospective survey of a varied collection of different case reports.

Cutting (1987) compared the PSE-rated symptomatology of 74 cases of organic

TABLE 3. *Comparison between abnormal and normal CT scan groups.*

	Abnormal scan	Normal scan	Significant difference at 95% probability*
Number	41	166	
Males, No. (%)	30 (73%)	111 (67%)	ns
Mean age at scan, years (SD)	35.2 (± 14.2)	32.5 (± 11.5)	ns
Mean age at first psychiatric contact (SD)	26.0 (± 10.6)	24.8 (± 7.7)	ns
Family history in first degree relative of treated:			
Schizophrenia or schizo-affective psychosis	1 (2%)	28 (17%)	$p = 0.033$
Manic depressive psychosis	1 (2%)	17 (10%)	ns
Unspecified psychosis	1(2%)	7 (4%)	ns
Suicide	2 (5%)	3 (2%)	ns
Other psychiatric disorder	4 (10%)	15 (9%)	ns
Family history in second degree relative of treated			
Schizophrenia or schizo- affective	2 (5%)	5 (3%)	ns
Manic depressive psychosis	2 (5%)	12 (7%)	ns
Unspecified psychosis	1 (2%)	17 (10%)	ns
Suicide	1 (2%)	6 (4%)	ns
Impaired premorbid personality	15 (37%)	22 (13%)	$p = 0.001$
First rank symptoms	146 (88%)	33 (80%)	ns
Formal thought disorder	21 (51%)	50 (30%)	$p = 0.018$
Mean number of prior admissions (SD)	3.24 (± 2.22)	3.31 (± 2.73)	ns
Mean percentage of time (between 1st contact and scan) spent as inpatient (SD)	25.7 (± 21.6)	24.6 (± 21.6)	ns
Mean number of previous non-schizophrenia discharge diagnoses per patient (SD)	0.59 (± 0.67)	0.31 (± 0.58)	$p = 0.010$
Interval in months between first contact and first discharge with diagnosis of schizophrenia mean (SD)	34.2 (± 59)	13.9 (± 33)	$p = 0.003$
EEG abnormal, with number tested (per cent)	14/33 (42%)	13/113 (12%)	$p = 0.0002$

*Test used: Chi-squared with Yates' correction (DF=1)
two-tailed Student's t (DF=205)

psychosis with 74 cases of Research Diagnostic Criteria acute schizophrenia, all prospectively interviewed. Like Davison and Bagley he found auditory hallucinations to be less common in the organic group. Delusions were also less frequently found, although simple persecutory delusions were actually more common in the organic group. Contrary to the findings of Davison and Bagley, Schneiderian symptoms were rare in the organic group (3%). Thought disorder and visual hallucinations were more common. Cutting also noted a difference in the content of the phenomenology. Whereas delusions of the first rank were unusual in organic cases, in nearly one half of the deluded organic patients, two delusional themes were apparent: either belief of imminent misadventure to others, or bizarre occurrences in the immediate vicinity. Few non-organic schizophrenic patients showed these features. Cutting offers possible explanations for these organic themes as being delusional elaborations of deficits of perception, or memory. In the area of perceptual disturbance, the mistaken identity of other people was another theme found more commonly in the organic group.

In the study of Johnstone *et al.* (1988), a PSE-rated symptomatology was compared between 23 cases of organic psychosis and 92 non-organic psychoses matched for age, sex and ethnicity conforming to DSM-3 criteria for schizophrenia, mania and psychotic depression. The authors found considerable overlap in symptoms. Comparing the organic and schizophrenic ($n = 43$) groups, nuclear (first rank) schizophrenic symptoms tended to be less frequent in the organic group (50% versus 74%, $p < 0.06$). Visual hallucinations were more common in the organic group only if consciousness was clouded.

In the series of Research Diagnostic Criteria schizophrenia patients under 65 referred to in the previous section, Lewis (1987*a*) compared clinical features of those 41 patients with unequivocally abnormal CT scans to features in the 166 with a normal CT scan. Those with abnormal CT had significantly less evidence of a family history of schizophrenia in first degree relatives, were significantly more likely to have had an impairment of premorbid personality, were more likely to have demonstrated formal thought disorder, and more often had EEG abnormalities (Table 3). Clinical presentation also seemed more atypical in the abnormal scan group, in that these patients were significantly more likely to have received alternative prior discharge diagnosis and a longer interval had intervened before a diagnosis of schizophrenia was made.

Distinguishing Organic from Functional Psychosis: Practical Guidelines

From this review, it can be seen that there are practical pointers in the history and presentation of a patient with psychotic symptoms which should be followed in excluding organic causes. Neuropsychological assessment will be dealt with in the next section.

(i) *Personal History*
Neurodevelopmental risk factors which can give rise to static, longstanding brain lesions and schizophrenia should be sought.

(a) Obstetric complications; including adverse events in pregnancy (viral infection, pre-eclampsia, antepartum haemorrhage) as well as during delivery (long or arrested labour, emergency Caesarian, prolapsed cord, postmaturity). Standardized assessment using a reliable and valid instrument (Lewis *et al.*, 1989) is possible. The patient's mother is the best informant.

(b) Childhood neurological events: in particular encephalitis; head injury severe enough to warrant hospital admission.

(c) Developmental motor delays, including delayed speech and walking; squints; severe stammering; enuresis.

(d) Minor physical anomalies on examination, such as unusual facies; congenital malformations.

(ii) *Family History*

Organic psychoses can arise secondary to some inherited brain diseases. With autosomal dominant disorders, such as Huntington's disease, a family history is usual, although sporadic cases arising through new mutations are not uncommon. A family history of schizophrenia or affective disorder will support a diagnosis of uncomplicated functional psychosis in the proband.

(iii) *Past Medical History*

Epilepsy; head injury; syphilis; intracranial infections; thyroid disorder; SLE; sarcoidosis; multiple sclerosis; HIV infection. All these can be complicated by an organic psychosis. In HIV disease, mania seems to be more common than is schizophrenia-like psychosis, although both can occur. Steroids can give mania or less commonly a paranoid psychosis.

(iv) *Drug and Alcohol History*

Short-lived paranoid psychoses can arise after cannabis misuse in susceptible persons, hallucinogen misuse, and misuse of amphetamines (including "ecstasy") and cocaine. Visual and tactile ("fornication" with cocaine) hallucinations are common. Sudden withdrawal from high-dose benzodiazepines can cause brief psychotic phenomena. Alcoholic hallucinosis occurs only in the context of longstanding dependence.

(v) *Symptoms and Mental State*

The following clinical symptoms and signs should prompt a search for organic aetiologies:

(a) Catatonic features

(b) Visual or tactile or olfactory hallucinations

(c) Delusions of particular themes: delusional misidentification; delusions of imminent danger to others; delusions of bizarre occurrences in the immediate vicinity.

(d) Atypical schizophrenia-like psychoses without first-rank symptoms or negative symptoms.

(e) Subtle disturbance in level of consciousness, e.g. perplexity.

TABLE 4. *Table of recommended screening procedures.*

Physical Investigations

First Line	Second Line
Neurological Examination	Auto Antibodies
Full Blood Count	CT Scan
ESR	Serum Calcium
Electrolytes	HIV
Syphilis Serology	Arysulphatase A
Thyroid Function	Karyotype
Liver Function	Chromosome studies
EEG	Serum Copper studies
Urinary Drug Screen	CSF examination

Neuropsychological Testing
Below is listed a brief representative sample of some of the tests which may be used. For each test the specific neurological impairment being assessed is briefly described.

1. Pre-morbid level of functioning
National Adult Reading Test   – to provide an estimate of premorbid
(Nelson and Willison, 1991)   ability as a comparative measure.

2. Current level of intellectual functioning
Wechsler Adult Intelligence Scale – Revised
(Wechsler, 1981)   – to provide a measure of current
                                              intellectual functioning.

3. Memory
Material or modality specific memory tasks related to temporal lobe functioning.

Wechsler Memory Scale – Revised
(Wechsler, 1987)   – to assess memory for verbal and figural
                                              stimuli, meaningful and abstract material
                                              and delayed as well as immediate recall.

Rey Auditory Verbal Learning Test
(Rey, 1964)   – assesses deficits of new verbal learning.

Recognition Memory Test
(Warrington, 1984)   – tests verbal and visual memory separately.

Benton Visual Retention Test
(Benton, 1974)   – test of visual recall thought to be better
                                              than some other tests in distinguishing
                                              patients with brain damage from those
                                              with psychiatric disorders (Marsh and
                                              Hirsch, 1982).

TABLE 4 (continued). *Table of recommended screening procedures*

Language
Graded Naming Test
(McKenna and Warrington, 1983)   – naming deficits.

Token Test
(De Renzi and Vignolo, 1962)   – comprehension deficits.

Spatial and Perceptual Abilities
related to parietal lobe function.

Rey Figure (copy) (Rey, 1959)   – Visuo-spatial, visuo-constructional deficits.

WAIS-R – Block Design   On Rey Figure
WAIS-R – Object Assembly   psychiatric patients differ from brain
                                       damaged patients in that they have been
                                       found to add bizarre embellishments to their
                                       drawings.

Executive Functions
Tests of abstraction, conceptual skills and planning related to frontal lobe function.

Modified Wisconsin Card Sorting Test
(Nelson, 1976)   – Rigidity of thinking, perseveration.

Verbal Fluency Test
(Benton *et al.*, 1983)

Design Fluency
(Jones, Gotman and Milner, 1977)   – Perseveration

Trail Making Test (Reiten, 1966)   – Lack of mental flexibility and control
                                       of inhibition. Sensitive to presence of
                                       brain damage. However, diagnostic
                                       differentiation between brain damage and
                                       psychiatric patients not consistent
                                       (Heaton *et al.*, 1978).

Physical Investigations

Table 4 outlines first- and second-line physical investigations in new cases of psychosis. Of the first-line investigations, some may dispute the need always for syphilis serology and EEG. However, a dozen or so cases of GPI present annually in the UK. The EEG is looking for generalized slowing indicative of diffuse brain disease, or the focal paroxysmal spike-and-wave discharges of an epileptic focus. The second-line investigations are dependent on other abnormal findings (autoantibodies if raised ESR, chromosome studies if developmental delays or unusual morphology). In particular, CT scan is only warranted in clinical practice if there are neurological symptoms in the history (e.g. epilepsy), or neurological signs on examination, or with an abnormal EEG.

Neuropsychology

Theoretically, the neuropsychological identification of an organic component in a psychotic illness should rely on the same criteria as are used to determine whether neurotic complaints have an organic aetiology. In these cases, a pattern of intellectual dysfunction selectively involving predominantly lateralized abilities and skills make a strong case for organicity, as does an organic pattern of memory impairment in which recent memory is more severely affected than remote memory, or a pattern of lowered scores on tests involving attention functions and new learning relative to scores on tests of knowledge and skill. Inconsistent or erratic expressions of cognitive defects on tests of intellectual function, language and memory would be more suggestive of a functional disturbance.

Identifying those psychotic conditions that have an organic component is often more difficult than distinguishing neurotic conditions or character disorders from symptoms of brain damage. Recent studies of brain dysfunction in schizophrenia have yielded evidence of neuropsychological and psychophysiological dysfunctions, as well as biochemical and structural abnormalities (Snyder, 1982; Weinberger et al.,1983; Holzman, 1985).

It is for this reason that the empirical battery approach based on quantitative summary scores does not discriminate well between brain-damaged and schizophrenic/psychotic patients. Functional impairment associated with attitudinal, attentional and motivational deficits in psychosis and impairment associated with structural loss or damage are difficult to differentiate on the basis of quantitative data. Differentiation often relies more on qualitative analysis of error patterns and performance styles rather than the exclusive reliance on test scores and levels of overall performance (Milberg et al., 1986; Weiss and Seidman, 1988). In addition, the assumption that schizophrenics should differ from certain neurological patients may be incorrect, given the hypothesis of underlying brain pathophysiology in this disorder.

Research on neuropsychological functioning in schizophrenia has raised a number of issues which serve to complicate the interpretation of neuropsychological test results. First, the question of generalized deficit in schizophrenia should be taken into account. As schizophrenic patients perform poorly on many cognitive tasks it is difficult to determine which deficits have aetiological significance and which are due to non-specific generalized factors. This distinction is especially difficult to make if performance is assessed by test scores rather than by response style and error patterns.

Secondly, the variable and extended course of schizophrenic illness means that changes in clinical state and deterioration in function must be taken into account to determine which deficits are state or trait related and this requires repeated assessment of patients over time. Therefore duration and severity of illness as well as clinical state are important factors. Impaired performance on tests is more characteristic of chronic than of acute schizophrenia (Golden *et al.*, 1983).

Thirdly, the effects of medication and treatment, including hospitalization must be considered. With respect to medication it may be argued that many neuro-psychological findings, particularly those relating to frontal, attentional, and executive functions may at least be partly due to treatment with neuroleptic drugs (Goldberg, 1985).

Fourthly, it should be borne in mind that attempts to localize brain dysfunction in schizophrenia from neuropsychological test performance are often based on comparisons with adult neurological patients. The brain dysfunction in schizo-phrenia however is likely to be developmental and the resulting pattern of deficits may therefore be different from adult onset lesions.

Lastly, the heterogeneity of schizophrenia is likely to be relevant, in that, different patterns of symptoms probably show different deficits on testing. Patients with CT abnormalities are more likely to have impairments on testing (see above).

Utility of Neuropsychological Tests
Schizophrenic patients have been noted to display various deficits on neuro-psychological tests which should be borne in mind when attempting to use them for the purposes of differential diagnosis. As psychiatric illness can disrupt attentional, perceptual and thinking skills as severely as those observed in patients with organic conditions, a lowered test score is not as reliable an indicator of organicity as when observed in another non-psychiatric patient. One needs therefore to have a clear cut pattern of lateralized dysfunction or organic memory impairment or a number of signs before concluding that brain damage may be present.

Premorbid Level of Functioning
Tests such as the National Adult Reading Test (Nelson and Willison, 1991) provide an indication of premorbid intellectual ability which can be compared with current levels of functioning to ascertain if and how much deterioration has occurred (see Chapter 7 for details). A review of the literature (Aylward *et al.*, 1984) concludes that although premorbid IQ in schizophrenic patients may be lower than would be expected from family and environmental variables, it does not appear to drop before the overt appearance of schizophrenic symptoms.

Current Level of Intellectual Functioning
Current level of intellectual functioning is usually assessed by the Wechsler Adult Intelligence Scale Scale – Revised (WAIS-R) (see Chapter 7 for details). Various studies comparing the performance of schizophrenic patients with brain damaged patients on the WAIS (Wechsler, 1958; Chelune *et al.*, 1979) have found that

although both groups are characterized by higher Verbal IQ than Performance IQ no specific pattern of subtest performance distinguishes them. In these cases an examination of qualitative evidence including unevenness of response, bizarre or symbolic responses suggestive of thought disorder or absence of patterns usually found in the performance of organically impaired patients observed during the course of one's own clinical experience may be helpful in further differentiating the two. For example, on the Vocabulary subtest of the WAIS-R patients with thought disorders sometimes reveal a thinking problem by "clangy" expressions, or idiosyncratic or bizarre associations, in contrast to limited responses associated with organic conditions such as dysphasia. On the Similarities subtest, which tests abstract concept formation, organically impaired patients often respond with differences, despite being corrected by the examiner. Unusual responses on the other hand are most often made by psychiatric patients.

Memory

Deficits of retention, recall and new learning of verbal or visual material are characteristic of organic memory problems. For example, the disassociation between old and new associate pairs on a learning task of the Wechsler Memory Scale (the Paired Associates task) is consistent with organic amnesia. A differential deficit of recall as compared with recognition tasks, together with evidence for poor clustering, suggests that verbal memory deficits in schizophrenia may be related to poor organizational skills in the encoding phase (Perlick et al. 1986). This pattern also suggests that attention and motivation contribute to schizophrenic patients' difficulty with verbal recall (see Chapter 7 for details of some commonly used memory test).

Attention

Attention deficits appear frequently in clinical descriptions of the schizophrenic syndrome (Kraeplin, 1919; Bleuler, 1950). Non-paranoid and negative symptom schizophrenia patients perform more poorly on tests of attention than do paranoid or positive symptom patients. An impairment of attention is widely accepted both as a clinical symptom and as an underlying mechanism of other cognitive dysfunctions in schizophrenia. One theory suggests that schizophrenics are unable to attend selectively to incoming stimuli (Neuchterlein and Dawson, 1984). Further, attentional deficits may be related to a generalized slowing of cognitive functions in schizophrenia (Gjerde, 1983).

Motor Control

One consistent finding in studies of psycho-motility in schizophrenics is a slowing in response speed (Goldstein, 1986). A possible confounding variable is attention. However, several studies using pure motor measures have reported significantly slowed bilateral motor responses in schizophrenic subjects. A slowed motor response would therefore not appear to be secondary to, though it is related to, cognitive attentional function.

Language

There is little evidence for impairment of basic language functions such as naming, repetition and simple syntax in schizophrenic patients (Morice and McNicol, 1986). Studies of language functions which have found impairment in semantic content and complex language suggest these are related to problems with attention or executive functions.

Spatial Abilities

Visuo-constructional deficits have been identified in some schizophrenic patients. They are, however, not consistent with impairment of primary visuo-perceptual processes, but more to do with organizational and executive dysfunctions. The observation of intact simple perceptual and constructional abilities is consistent with Kolb and Whishaw's (1983) findings of normal performance on tests of parietal function, e.g. copying (Rey figure).

Executive Functions

Executive functions are cognitive processes that allow the subject to respond and adapt appropriately to his or her environment (Walsh, 1985). From a neuro-psychological point of view, executive functions have been described as the ability to get into the appropriate response set for a given task, to maintain that set, and to shift the set as needed. Therefore schizophrenics are consistently impaired on tests of executive function with demonstrated sensitivity to frontal lesions (e.g. Wisconsin Card Sorting Test, Word Fluency, Gottman Design Fluency Test). In fact, with the possible exception of temporal lobe epilepsy, it is frontal lobe dysfunction more than any other focal neurological condition which can be confused diagnostically with schizophrenia.

There are certain behavioural deficits commonly observed in some frontal lobe patients and some schizophrenic patients, i.e. perseveration and "memory-like" deficits. In frontal patients, verbal recall deficits are executive in nature, i.e. there is an inability to subordinate selectively the process of retrieval. Instead, the process of recall takes on the quality of a chain of free associations which are not subjected to editing by either the context of the task or the material to be recalled. This is similar to certain aspects of cognitive deficits seen in schizophrenia both with respect to perseveration and particularly with respect to the structure of "un-edited" associative responses to certain verbal and conceptual tasks.

In spite of the fact that their performance on a limited number of tests sensitive to the executive deficit might appear similar, in the case of frontal pathology due to distinct neurological condition (tumour, trauma, aneurysm, etc.) this breakdown of hierarchical organization of behaviour is superimposed on a premorbidly fully formed completed pattern of hierarchic organization; what is observed is genuinely a breakdown. In certain forms of schizophrenia at least, it seems likely that the whole course of cognitive development is affected long before the first overt psychotic symptom manifests itself. This is therefore a maldevelopment of the hierarchical organization of behaviour rather than the breakdown of one that was once intact, i.e. the "depth of deficits" is presumed greater in schizophrenia than in focal frontal pathology of later onset.

Illustrative Clinical Case Reports

The following cases help to illustrate that both false positives and false negatives are possible. The developmental lesion in Case 1 showed no neuropsychological sequelae, whereas the acquired lesion in Case 2 did – most particularly, a subtle visuo-spatial amnesic deficit which probably related to the observed psychiatric symptoms.

Case 1
A 55-year-old man had a 25-year history of relapsing psychosis with a clinical diagnosis of paranoid schizophrenia. His mother had a well documented history of manic-depressive psychosis. His childhood and early developmental history was unremarkable and his pre-morbid personality was good, with stable friendships and a good work history. There is no history of significant medical disorder. At age 30 he suffered an acute onset of persecutory delusions and third person auditory hallucinations in clear consciousness and in the absence of depressed mood. His symptoms resolved over a period of a month with chlorpromazine and he returned to his job 6 weeks later. There were five relatively brief hospital admissions during the next 5 years with one delusion of reference remaining stable over several years independently of acute relapses.

At interview he had been free of psychotic symptoms for 10 years and there was little evidence of a defect state. Neurological examination was unremarkable; he is left-handed and left-footed. Neuropsychological investigation revealed a WAIS Verbal IQ of 75, Performance 93. A Schonell Reading test showed a reading age of 7 years. CT and MRI scans showed complete agenesis of the corpus callosum with a left sided fronto-temporal cyst. Tests of bimanual motor coordination and inter-hemispheric transfer of tacile and visual information were given. No deficits emerged in comparison with two men of the same age with diagnoses of schizophrenia who had normal CT scans (from Lewis *et al.*, 1988).

Case 2
A 30-year-old man had his first psychotic episode whose form was a subacute confusional state with paranoid symptoms. His elder sister had had two psychiatric admissions, although no details were available. The patient had an unremarkable childhood, and developmental milestones were normal. His premorbid personality was good. He was homosexual and 6 months prior to the psychiatric symptoms he developed opportunistic infections and received a diagnosis of AIDS. Psychiatric symptoms followed the onset of pneumocystis pneumonia with resulting hypoxia. For several days he developed the fixed belief that friends who visited had been replaced by alien imposters who were physically identical, but actually working with the IRA. These imposters had abducted him to a place which resembled a

hospital ward but in reality was a room in a garage. He also experienced visual and auditory hallucinations in the third person. These psychotic phenomena lasted for a week and improved with haloperidol. Neurological examination was normal and urine drug screen negative. CT scan at this time showed a small area of low density in the right upper medial parietal region thought to be compatible with a pneumocystis lesion. Neurological testing performed 3 weeks after the psychotic symptoms had resolved showed WAIS-R Verbal and Performance IQs showing a significant decline from 113 and 110 respectively premorbidly, to 109 and 94. Verbal memory was intact and immediate recall of simple designs was normal. However, there was a specific visuo-spatial deficit for recall of patterns not available for verbal coding; in particular, recognition memory for faces was borderline. Perceptual and naming skills and frontal lobe tests were normal.

References

Aylward, E. *et al.* (1984). Intelligence in schizophrenia: meta analysis of the research. *Schizophrenia Bulletin,* **10**, 430-459.

Benton, A.L. (1955). "The Visual Retention Test". The Psychological Corporation, New York.

Benton, A.L. and Hamshen, K. de S., Varney, N.R., and Spreen, O. (1983). "Contributions to Neuropsychological Assessment". Oxford University Press, New York.

Bleuler, E. (1950). "The Group of Schizophrenics". (Ed. J. Zinkin, Trans) International University Press (Original work published 1911), New York.

Coughlan, A.K. and Hollows, S.E. (1985). "The Adult Memory and Information Processing Battery". (Ed. A.K. Coughlan).

Crichton, P. and Lewis, S.W. (1990). Delusional misidentification, AIDS and the right hemisphere. *British Journal of Psychiatry,* in press.

Cummings, J.L. (1985). Organic delusions: Phenomenology, anatomical correlations and review. *British Journal of Psychiatry,* **146**, 184-189.

Cutting, J. (1987). The phenomenology of acute organic psychosis: comparison with acute schizophrenia. *British Journal of Psychiatry,* **151**, 324-332.

Davison, K. and Bagley, C.R. (1969). Schizophrenia-like psychoses associated with organic disorders of the central nervous system. *In* "Current Problems in Neuropsychiatry: Schizophrenia, Epilepsy, the Temporal Lobe". (Ed. R. Herrington), London, *British Journal of Psychiatry* (Special publication No 4.)

De Renzi, E. and Vignolo, L.A. (1962). The Token Test; a sensitive test to detect receptive disturbances in aphasics. *Brain,* **85**, 665-678.

Gjerde, P.F. (1983). Attentional capacity dysfunction and arousal in schizophrenia. *Psychological Bulletin,* **93**, 57-72.

Eisenson, J. (1954). "Examining for Aphasia". Psychological Corporation, New York.

Goldberg, (1985). Akinesia, tardive dysmentia, and frontal lobe disorder in schizophrenia. *Schizophrenia Bulletin,* **11**, 255-263.

Golden, C.J., Carpenter, B. Wilkenny, G., Ruedrich, S., Chu, C. and Graber, B. (1983). The relationship of the Brief Psychiatric Rating Scale neuropsychological defects in phenomenologically treated schizophrenia. *Psychopharmacology Bulletin,* **19**, 513-512.

Goldstein, G. (1986). The neuropsychology of schizophrenia. *In* "Neuropsychological

Assessment of Neuropsychiatric Disorders". (Eds I. Grant and K.M. Adams), pp. 147-171). Oxford University Press, New York.

Goldstein, K. and Scheerer, M. (1941). Abstract and concrete behaviour: an experimental study with special tests. *Psychological Monographs*, **43**, 1-151.

Goodglass, H. and Kaplan, E. (1972). "The Assessment of Aphasia and Related Disorders". Lea and Febiger, Philadelphia.

Heaton, R.K., Baade, L.E., and Johnson, K.L. (1978). Neuropsychological test results associated with psychiatric disorders in adults. *Psychological Bulletin*, **85**, 141-162.

Holzman, P.S. (1985). Eye movement dysfunction and psychosis. *International Review of Neurobiology*, **27**, 179-205.

Johnstone, E. *et al.* (1988). Phenomenology of organic and functional psychoses and the overlap between them. *British Journal of Psychiatry*, **153**, 770-776.

Jones-Gotman, M. and Milner, B. (1977). Design fluency – the production of nonesense drawings after focal cortical lesions. *Neuropsychologica*, **15**, 653-674.

Kolb, B. and Whishaw, I.Q. (1983). Performance of schizophrenic patients on tests sensitive to left or right frontal, temporal or parietal function in neurological patients. *Journal of Nervous and Mental Diseases*, **171**, 435-443.

Kraeplin, E. (1919). "Dementia Praecox and Paraphrenia". (Ed. R.M. Barclay, Trans). E. and S. Livingstone (Original work published 1913), Edinburgh.

Kuhnley, E.J., White, D.H. and Granoff, A.L. (1981). Psychiatric presentation of arachoid cyst. *Journal of Clinical Psychiatry*, **42**, 167-169.

Levin, S. and Yurgelvn Todd, D. (1989). Contributions of clinical neuropsychology to the study of schizophrenia. *Journal of Abnormal Psychology*, **98**, No. 4, 341-356.

Lewis, S.W. (1987). Schizophrenia with and without abnormal intracranial morphology. M.Phil Thesis, University of London.

Lewis, S.W. (1989). Congenital risk factors for schizophrenia. *Psychological Medicine*, **19**, 5-13.

Lewis, S.W. and Mezey, G.C. (1985). Clinical correlates of septum pellucidum cavities: an unusual association with psychosis. *Psychological Medicine*, **15**, 43-54.

Lewis, S. W., Reveley, A.M., Reveley, M.A., Chitkara, B. and Murray, R.M. (1987). The familial-sporadic distinction in schizophrenia research. *British Journal of Psychiatry*, **151**, 306-313.

Lewis, S.W., Revely, M.A., David, A.S. and Ron, M.A. (1988). Agenesis of the corpus callosum and schizophrenia. *Psychological Medicine*, **18**, 341-347.

Lishman, W.A. (1987). "Organic Psychiatry".

Marsh, G.G. and Hirsch, S.H. (1982). Effectiveness of two tests of visual retention. *Journal of Clinical Psychology*, **38**, 115-118.

McKenna, P. and Warrington, E.K. (1980). Testing for nominal dysphasia. *Journal of Neurology, Neurosurgery and Psychiatry*, **43**, 781-88.

Milberg, W., Hebben, N. and Kaplan, E. (1986). The Boston process approach to neurospsychological assessment. *In* "Neuropsychological Assessment of Neuropsychiatric Disorders". (Eds I.Grant and K.M. Adam), pp. 65-86. Oxford University Press, New York.

Morice, R.D. (1986). Beyond language – speculations on the pre-frontal cortex and schizophrenia. *Australian and New Zealand Journal of Psychiatry*, **20**, 7-10.

Morice, R.D. and McNicol, D. (1986). Language changes in schizophrenia: a limited replication. *Schizophrenia Bulletin*, **12**, 239-251.

Moses, J.A. Cardinello, J.P. and Thompson, L.L. (1983). Discrimination of brain damage from chronic psychosis by the Luria-Nebraska neuropsychological battery. A closer look. *Journal of Consulting and Clinical Psychology,* **51**, 441-449.

Nelson, H.E. (1976). A modified card sorting test sensitive to frontal lobe deficits, *Cortex,* **12**, 313-324. ·

Nelson, H.E. and O'Connell, A. (1978). Dementia: the estimation of premorbid intelligence levels using the new adult reading test. *Cortex,* **14**, 234-244.

Nelson, N.E. and Willion, J. (1991). "Natural Adult Reading Test (NART)". 2nd Edn. NFER – Nelson.

Owens, D.G.C. Johnstone, E.C., Bydder, G.M. and Kreel, L. (1980). Unsuspected organic disease in chronic schizophrenia demonstrated by computed tomography. *Journal of Neurology, Neurosurgery and Psychiatry,* **43**, 1065-1069.

Perlick, D., Stastny, P., Katz, I., Mayer, M. and Mattis, S. (1986). Memory deficits and anticholinergic levels in chronic schizophrenia. *American Journal of Psychiatry,* **143**, 230-232.

Ravens, J.C. (1976). "Manual for Raven's Progressive Matrices and Vocabulary Scales". H.K. Lewis, London.

Reitan, R.M. (1964). Psychological deficits resulting from cerebral lesions in man. *In* "The Frontal Granular Cortex and Behaviour". (Eds J.M. Warren and K. Akert). Ch. 14. McGraw Hill, New York.

Rey, A. (1959). "Le Test de copie de Figure complexe". Editions Centre de Psychologie appliquée, Paris.

Rey, A. (1964). "l'Examen clinique en Psychologie". Presses Universitaires de France, Paris.

Snyder, S.M. (1982). Neurotransmittors and CNS disease: Schizophrenia. *Lancet,* **2**, 970-974.

Walsh, K.W. (1985). "Understanding Brain Damage: a Primer of Neuropsychological Evaluation". Churchill Livingstone, New York.

Warrington, E.K. (1984). "Recognition Memory Test". NFER. Nelson.

Wechsler, D. (1987). Wechsler Memory Scale – Revised. The Psychological Corporation.

Wechsler, D. (1981). "Manual for the Wechsler Adult Intelligence Scale - Revised". The Psychological Corporation, New York.

Weinberger, D.R., Wagner, R.L. and Wyatt, R.J. (1983). Neuropathological studies in schizophrenia: a selective review. *Schizophrenia Bulletin,* **9**, 193.

Weiss, J.L. and Seidman, L.J. (1988). The clinical use of psychological test. *In* "The New Harvard Guide to Psychology". pp. 46-69. Belknap Press of Harvard University Press, Cambridge, MA.

World Health Organisation (1978). Mental Disorders: ICD. WHO, Geneva.

13. Assessment of Movement Disorder in Psychosis

Thomas R.E. Barnes and John M. Kane

The Assessment of Drug-Induced Movement Disorders

Patients treated with antipsychotic (neuroleptic) drugs for psychotic illness may exhibit a broad range of abnormal involuntary movements. The acute problems are parkinsonism, acute akathisia and acute dystonia, while the chronic conditions are tardive dystonia, chronic akathisia and tardive dyskinesia. The characteristic features of these conditions, some of the problems in their assessment and the clinical utility of selected rating scales are presented here.

Tardive dyskinesia, particularly, is often seen as a major constraint upon the long-term administration of neuroleptics. Aetiological explanations for tardive dyskinesia refer to the effects of medication, manifestations of the psychotic illness, or an interaction between the drug treatment and the psychotic disease process. However, prospective studies in psychiatric patients treated with antipsychotic drugs suggest that the incidence of tardive dyskinesia increases with increasing exposure to medication, arguing for some aetiological role for drug treatment, precipitating if not producing the movement disorder. Clinical investigation of these issues is hampered by the lack of availability of a control group of psychotic patients who have not received antipsychotic medication during their illness. Patients with psychotic illness almost invariably have a history of exposure to antipsychotic medication, and an observer attempting to evaluate and rate abnormal movements must be aware that both drug-related and illness-related movements may be present in an individual patient. While the drug-induced movements have been classified into a number of relatively discrete syndromes, the movements described as occurring as an inherent part of the psychotic illness cover a wide range of phenomena, from a lack of co-ordination, simple tic-like disturbances and grimacing to chorea (Marsden et al., 1975; Casey and Hansen, 1984). The rating scales for abnormal involuntary movements currently available tend to avoid any attempt to discriminate between movements that might be illness-related and those which are drug-induced. However, the latter aetiology is usually assumed when rating the recognized phenomena of syndromes such as parkinsonism, akathisia and acute dystonia.

Another problem in the assessment of abnormal involuntary movements is that they are influenced by the patient's degree of arousal. Thus, the circumstances of the assessment can influence the severity of the condition. If the patient feels stressed or agitated the condition is often exacerbated while the movements may be ameliorated if the patient is relaxed or sedated, and absent during sleep. Nevertheless, the systematic and reliable assessment of the drug-induced movement disorders is essential in both research and clinical settings. In research, the ability to reliably measure these conditions both quantitatively and qualitatively is necessary for treatment studies, for the evaluation of the side-effect profiles of antipsychotic drugs and for the investigation of the relationships between the various movement disorders and relevant clinical variables. Clinically, rating instruments can be a diagnostic aid and allow more systematic monitoring of movement disorders during individual therapeutic trials.

The Assessment Procedures

Parkinsonism

Signs of drug-induced parkinsonism may develop within days of starting antipsychotic medication. According to the literature, the incidence in routine clinical practice seems to vary widely, with figures up to 40%. The condition resembles idiopathic Parkinson's disease in many respects, the main phenomena being muscle rigidity, tremor, postural abnormalities and bradykinesia. However, some authors have commented that some of the characteristic features of the idiopathic condition, such as the festinant, hurrying gait and 3-5 Hz, resting tremor are not so common in drug-induced parkinsonism (Schwab and England, 1968; Hershey *et al.*, 1982).

Perhaps the most typical sign of the drug-induced condition is rigidity of the limbs, best tested by passive movement of a patient's limbs. The examiner may experience a sustained resistance, referred to as "lead pipe" rigidity, or a succession of resistances that are rapidly overcome, known as "cog-wheel" rigidity. During such an examination, patients may find it hard to relax and allow their limbs to be moved passively. If an examiner is uncertain about the presence of rigidity in a limb, the technique of activation may be useful. When the subject is asked to actively move the opposite limb, the rigidity in the arm being tested tends to become more obvious. The assessment may also be confused by the patient's voluntary movements. For example, a patient may move a limb in synchrony with the examiner's passive movements or resist the movements. This problem can be partly countered by the examiner carrying out the passive movements in an unpredictable way, switching from joint to joint and varying the speed.

Extrapyramidal Side-effects Rating Scale (EPSE)
(Simpson and Angus, 1970)

The Extrapyramidal side-effects (EPSE) rating scale developed by Simpson and Angus (1970) is the most popular of the available scales. It was devised to measure drug-induced parkinsonism, providing standardized clinical assessment of rigidity, tremor and salivation. It consists of 10 items, each rated on a five-point scale (0-4).

Reliability and validity

Simpson and Angus (1970) attempted to validate the scale by demonstrating that it effectively separated three groups of patients receiving different doses of antipsychotic medication. They also measured the inter-rater reliability of the scale items. In a sample of 14 patients examined on two occasions by two doctors, virtually all items achieved an acceptable level of agreement, although ratings on the rigidity items tended to show the highest correlation coefficients between the raters. The mean correlation coefficients ranged from 0.87 for glabella tap and 0.78 for shoulder shaking to 0.56 for the tremor item and 0.52 for gait. Correlations between the two raters on the total scale scores ranged from 0.71 to 0.96

Utility

Perhaps the main disadvantage of the scale is that it is not particularly comprehensive in the symptoms and signs measured, being heavily weighted on items rating rigidity. Seven of the 10 scale items measure rigidity, such as arm dropping, shoulder shaking, elbow rigidity and wrist rigidity. However, a scale devised by Webster (1968) for rating Parkinson's disease, also has 10 items, but only one refers to rigidity. The other items rate bradykinesia, parkinsonian posture, arm swing, gait, tremor, facies, seborrhoea, speech and self care. Although designed for assessment of the idiopathic condition, it has been employed in studies of drug-induced parkinsonism (Casey *et al.*, 1980).

The recommended procedure for assessing neck rigidity is that the patient "lies on a well-padded examining table and his head is raised by the examiner's hand. The hand is then withdrawn and the head allowed to drop. In the normal subject the head will fall upon the table. The movement is delayed in extrapyramidal system disorder, and in extreme parkinsonism it is absent." The main problem with this procedure is that it tends to work only once. On subsequent testing, when the element of surprise is lost, patients tend to keep their heads up after the examiner's hand is withdrawn so as to avoid it hitting the table. The differential diagnosis might also include the "invisible pillow" sign, seen as a feature of catatonic schizophrenia.

The EPSE has only one item for tremor. A rating of 1 or 2 refers to observed tremor of the fingers and arm, and whole body tremor is necessary to obtain a maximum score. There is no separate rating for signs such as head tremor (titubation) or tongue tremor. Tremor is a protean symptom and a rater may experience difficulties discriminating between minimal parkinsonian tremor, tremor related to anxiety or medication such as lithium, and benign essential tremor. The EPSE recommends that the patient "is observed walking into the examining room and then re-examined for this item." This suggests that it is observable resting tremor that is being rated, rather than postural tremor elicited by a specific examination procedure. However, postural tremor is relatively common in psychiatric patients on medication and if taken by a rater as a sign of parkinsonism could inflate the score on this item quite dramatically compared with a rate limiting the rating to resting tremor.

Pooling of saliva in the mouth is another feature of drug-induced parkinsonism.

The relevant EPSE item rates salivation from normal (scoring 0) to "Speaking with difficulty because of excess salivation" (3), and most severely, "Frank drooling" (4). One explanation for this sign is that saliva accumulates in the mouth because the patient is swallowing less frequently than usual. However, hypersalivation can occur with antipsychotic drugs, unrelated to obvious parkinsonism. While this problem is uncommon with conventional antipsychotic drugs, and the mechanism is unclear, it occurs in approximately a third of patients receiving the recently introduced "atypical" antipsychotic, clozapine.

The Simpson and Angus scale does not include a rating for bradykinesia, or akinesia, a component of drug-induced parkinsonism that is characterized by features such as a lack of facial expression, paucity of gesture, a mask-like facies and slow monotonous speech. These features may be mistaken for retarded depression, so-called "akinetic depression", and there is also a potential overlap between these symptoms and negative features of schizophrenia such as affective flattening, poverty of speech and lack of drive (see Chapter 5).

The EPSE was published 20 years ago, and a modified version was presented by Mindham in 1976. One of the changes from the original is the inclusion of an item for lack of facial expression. This may be particularly liable to be confounded by lack of facial expression related to flattened affect. Other investigators (Rifkin *et al.*, 1978; Kane *et al.*, 1983) have utilized modified versions of the EPSE to include items for akinesia and akathisia.

Comparative utility
The emphasis on rigidity in the EPSE is a disadvantage if a comprehensive assessment of the phenomena of drug-induced parkinsonism is desired, but could possibly be an advantage if an objective measure is required that will not be confounded by the presence of negative symptoms such as flattened affect.

The major differences between the EPSE and the Mindham modification is that the latter allows for ratings of lateralized signs, and possesses an additional item for the global rating of parkinsonism. This "Global assessment of physical state" may present some difficulty for monitoring change in the severity of parkinsonism as a score of 3 refers to both moderate and severe parkinsonism. However, such a global rating may seem less arbitrary than the convention for calculating the global score for the EPSE, which involves adding all the item ratings and dividing by the total number of items. Simpson and Angus considered that a final score of up to 0.3 was "within the normal range".

Acute Dystonia

Acute dystonic reactions are involuntary movements dominated by sustained muscle contraction causing contorting, twisting, repetitive movements or abnormal postures (Fahn *et al.*, 1987). Patients usually complain spontaneously, as the muscle spasms are invariably painful and distressing, and often frightening. Nevertheless, dystonic reactions are commonly misdiagnosed or misinterpreted as dissociative phenomena, malingering or even as misguided attempts to persuade doctors to prescribe anticholinergic agents.

The muscles of the head and neck are most commonly affected. Symptoms can include sustained contraction of the masticatory muscles (trismus), forceful, sustained eye closure (blepharospasm), facial grimacing, oculogyric spasm (characterized by a brief, fixed stare, followed by upward and lateral rotation of the eyes so that only the sclera remain visible) dysarthria, dysphagia, glossopharyngeal contractions and torticollis. Abnormal movements of the limbs with dystonic arm movements or a dystonic gait are sometimes seen.

Until recently, acute dystonic reactions in patients receiving antipsychotic drugs were considered to be relatively rare, with a reported incidence of around 2-5% (Rupniak et al., 1986). However, a study by Addonzio and Alexopoulos (1988) suggested a much higher overall figure of 25%. Children and young adults are the most commonly affected. The reactions usually occur within a day or two of starting antipsychotic treatment, with the majority of cases occurring within 4 to 5 days of beginning the drugs (Ayd, 1961). Late onset, persistent dystonia, called tardive dystonia, is seen in patients on chronic antipsychotic treatment (Burke et al., 1982). Again, tardive dystonia was thought to be relatively uncommon, with a reported prevalence around 1.5 to 2% (Yassa et al., 1986). However, a recent detailed and systematic study (Sethi et al., 1990) using the Fahn-Marsden scale (see below), found a much higher prevalence.

Dystonia Movement Scale
(Burke et al., 1985)

No rating scale has been devised to specifically rate drug-induced dystonia. Perhaps this reflects that acute dystonic reactions are usually relatively transient phenomena, and respond rapidly to anticholinergic medication. However, Burke et al. (1985) have presented reliability and validity data on a scale for primary torsion dystonia called the Dystonia Movement Scale or the Fahn-Marsden scale which has been used for rating tardive dystonia. This scale is probably only appropriate for particularly severe, persistent cases of drug-induced dystonia.

This scale has two items rating provoking factors on a five-point scale (0-4): one is for the provocation of dystonia with activity, while the other refers specifically to speech and swallowing. The remaining items rat the severity of dystonia on a five-point scale at seven body regions: eyes, mouth, speech and swallowing, neck, arm, trunk and lag. Where appropriate, the severity ratings are partly based on functional disability. The total score is calculated by multiplying the severity score by the provoking factor score for each region, which yields a maximum score of 16 for each region except eyes, mouth and neck where the score is halved. Thus, the maximum total score on this scale is 120.

Akathisia

Akathisia is a syndrome of motor restlessness that is perhaps the most common and most distressing of all the drug-induced movement disorders (Barnes, 1987; Van Putten and Marder, 1987). The absence of established diagnostic criteria in the past, particularly the lack of delineation of the associated motor behaviour, may have been partly responsible for the wide range of prevalence figures reported, the failure of clinicians consistently to recognize the condition (Weiden *et al.*, 1987) and the common misdiagnosis of the motor phenomena of akathisia as signs and symptoms of psychiatric illness, such as an exacerbation of agitation or psychotic excitement (Van Putten and Marder, 1987).

Characteristically, patients with akathisia describe a subjective sense of inner restlessness, mental unease or dysphoria which can be intense. Typically, they also report that they are unable to keep their legs still or feel a compulsion to move. Many patients complain that the condition is least tolerable when they are required to stand still (Braude *et al.*, 1983). Also, patients with akathisia are sometimes aware of tension and discomfort in their limbs, with parasthesiae and unpleasant pulling or drawing sensations in their legs. These complaints are akin to symptoms found in the Restless Legs, or Ekbom's syndrome (Blom and Ekbom, 1961; Barnes, 1987). Diagnosis will involve specific enquiry to elicit the subjective experience of akathisia. Patients can be asked about the experience of inner restlessness, and whether they can locate restless, fidgety feelings to any part of their body. Symptoms referrable to the lower limbs seem to be the most characteristic (Braude *et al.*, 1983; Barnes and Braude, 1985). Further, patients can be asked if they have any awareness of restlessness and tension when required to stand still, or a compulsive desire to move.

However, reliance on subjective report alone may not be particularly reliable (Van Putten and Marder, 1986). The diagnosis also rests on the observation of characteristic movements that are not dyskinetic in nature but rather recognizable patterns of normal, restless movement. Perhaps the commonest movements associated with the subjective experience of akathisia are rocking from foot to foot and walking on the spot when standing (Braude *et al.*, 1983; Gibb and Lees, 1986). Seated patients with akathisia tend to shuffle or tramp their feet and swing one leg on the other. With severe akathisia, patients are unable to stand without walking or pacing. In addition to restless movements in the lower limbs, trunk rocking and fidgety movements of the upper limbs may be seen (Burke *et al.*, 1989; Walters *et al.*, 1989), although such movements are less typical of the syndrome (Braude *et al.*, 1983; Van Putten and Marder, 1987).

The motor phenomena of akathisia are more likely to be observed in naturalistic situations rather than during a formal interview. If patients are concentrating on some motor activity, or being physically examined, the movements may be suppressed. Nevertheless, akathisic movements can sometimes be effectively elicited by standing with the patient and engaging him in casual conversation.

Akathisia is recognized most commonly as an acute, dose-related side-effect of antipsychotic drugs. However, it may also occur as a chronic problem in patients on maintenance drug therapy (Barnes and Braude, 1985; Barnes, 1990) and in some cases may even persist after drug withdrawal (Weiner and Luby, 1983; Burke *et al.*, 1989). There are no obvious differences in the motor phenomena of acute and chronic akathisia although the accompanying subjective sense of restlessness in perhaps less marked in the latter.

For many years, systematic assessment of this condition was limited to isolated akathisia items from more general scales for extrapyramidal symptoms, such as the Chouinard Extrapyramidal Rating Scale (Chouinard *et al.*, 1980), the Hillside/LIJ modification of the Simpson and Angus (1970) Extrapyramidal Symptoms Scale (Adler *et al.*, 1989) and the Dimascio Reversible Extrapyramidal Symptom Scale (Dufresne and Wagner, 1988). Subjective and objective criteria for the condition were incorporated in some of the earlier akathisia scales (Bartels *et al.*, 1987; Friis *et al.*, 1982) although reliability data were not provided. A visual analogue scale, a 100 reliability data were not provided. A visual analogue scale, a 100 mm line with anchor points, has also been successfully employed in treatment studies (Adler *et al.*, 1986).

The use of a single scale item may be appropriate if akathisia is not the main focus of the movement disorder assessment. If more careful diagnosis and scrutiny of the akathisia syndrome is required, the scale used should allow for rating of both the subjective experience and the observable, restless movements.

Barnes Akathisia Rating Scale (BARS)
(Barnes, 1989)

The BARS comprises items for rating the observable, restless movements which characterize the condition, the subjective awareness of restlessness, and any distress associated with the akathisia. In addition, there is a global severity item, rating on a six-point (0-5) scale with operational definitions for each scale point. There is a recommended examination procedure. Each patient should be observed seated for at least 5 min. During the examination the patient should also be observed while remaining standing, engaged in informal conversation for several minutes. Symptoms noted while a patient is being observed in situations other than the interview and examination procedure may also be rated on the scale.

Specific questions about a subjective awareness of akathisia are best left to the end of the examination. Questioning about insomnia may be relevant as some patients are unable to get off to sleep because of the restlessness, and need to get out of bed and pace up and down.

Reliability and validity
Barnes (1989) reported the inter-rater reliability for the scale items, expressed in terms of linearly weighted Cohen's kappa, as ranging from 0.738 to 0.955, the

highest figure referring to the global item. The validity of this rating scale derives from its basis in the signs and symptoms found to be characteristic of the condition in clinical studies (Barnes and Braude, 1985; Braude *et al.*, 1983; Gibb and Lees, 1986; Van Putten and Marder, 1987).

Utility

The final item is a global clinical assessment and may be used alone as an overall severity measure. A rating of 2 or more is considered as diagnostic. In the absence of a rating on either of the two subjective items but a rating of 2 or 3 on the objective item, a patient would score 0 on the global item but be considered as a case of pseudoakathisia.

In mild cases of akathisia, the opposite situation is also found, where the signs of motor restlessness are not present despite a patient's description of the typical subjective experience. This has been referred to as "subjective akathisia" (Van Putten and Marder, 1986) and may be difficult to distinguish from subtle manifestations of anxiety or emotional distress unrelated to akathisia. This difficulty is acknowledged by the questionable rating (scoring 1) on the global item of the scale, and the existence of subjective akathisia is reflected in the mild (scoring 2) akathisia rating as it does not demand the presence of the characteristic restless movements.

The scale has been widely used, and is available in English, Italian and Japanese versions.

Hillside Akathisia Scale (HAS)
(Fleischhacker et al., 1989)

This scale also consists of subjective and objective items and a global item. The suggested examination procedure includes observation of patients while they are sitting, standing and lying down.

Reliability and validity

Reliability for rating subjective symptoms ranged from 0.86 to 0.92 and for objective ratings the figures ranged from 0.51 to 0.89. Reliability was 0.89 for the HAS total score and the correlation between the HAS and a global assessment of akathisia (modified CGI) was 0.87 (Fleischhaker *et al.*, 1992). As with all scales of akathisia, the major strategy for validation involves clinical application, for example, assessing medication effect, since there are no established biological or psychophysiological validating criteria.

Utility

The instrument was intended to be of use primarily in rating the severity of akathisia in clinical psychopharmacological research. Because of the diverse phenomenology of akathisia, movements are rated on the basis of frequency and severity. The instrument has been demonstrated to be sensitive to drug effects in clinical trials (Miller *et al.*, 1990) and is available in English and German versions.

Comparative utility

Both the BARS and HAS were developed specifically for assessing drug-induced akathisia. One advantage they both possess is the separate rating of subjective complaints and objective findings in akathisia, and the rating of the condition in both formal interview and more naturalistic settings.

In contrast to the BARS scale, the characteristic restless movements of akathisia to be rated on the HAS are not defined, and the rater decides whether the movements observed qualify as manifestations of akathisia.

Tardive Dyskinesia

The most characteristic and prevalent feature of this condition is orofacial dyskinesia. This refers to involuntary movements of the tongue, face, lips, jaw and face, including movements of the peri-orbital muscles. The movements described include protrusion or twisting of the tongue, smacking, pursing and sucking movements of the lips, puffing of the cheeks and chewing and lateral motion of the jaw. These movements are more obvious in edentulous patients, although in some cases the presence of dyskinesia may partly explain why they have not persisted with dentures.

In addition to these orofacial phenomena, most descriptions of tardive dyskinesia include a range of trunk and limb movements. The involuntary limb movements seen are purposeless, jerky and often rather stereotypic in nature, and usually described as choreiform or choreoathetoid. Athetosis of the extremities, and axial and limb dystonia are also included sometimes as part of the syndrome, as are grunting and respiratory arrhythmias and abnormalities of gait and trunk posture, such as lordosis, rocking and swaying, shoulder shrugging and rotary movements of the pelvis. There is evidence from several sources that orofacial and trunk and limb dyskinesia should be considered as distinct subsyndromes of tardive dyskinesia (Barnes, 1990; Inada *et al.*, 1990) and it may be appropriate to analyze ratings from the two regions separately.

Individual patients may show a wide variation in the site and severity of dyskinesia, related to alteration of medication such as change in dosage of antipsychotic or anticholinergic drugs, or changes in posture, mobility or level of physiological arousal. Also, apparently spontaneous fluctuations in the severity of the movements may occur from day to day or even within hours or minutes. This intra-patient variability is great enough to contribute to the likelihood of false negative assessments of tardive dyskinesia, particularly if patients are observed for only brief periods (Richardson *et al.*, 1982).

Spontaneous dyskinesia

Interpretation of data from rating scales for tardive dyskinesia must take into account the possible presence of spontaneous dyskinesia related to age or the schizophrenic illness. For example, so-called spontaneous or idiopathic orofacial dyskinesia, apparently indistinguishable from tardive dyskinesia, is seen in 1-15% of elderly individuals who have never received antipsychotic drugs (Blowers *et al.*,

1981; Kane *et al.*, 1982).

As mentioned above, motor disturbance related to the psychotic illness being treated may include disturbances of voluntary motor activity such as stereotypies, mannerisms, posturing (Marsden *et al.*, 1975) and choreiform and dystonic movements (Casey and Hansen, 1984). Such movements may appear identical to tardive dyskinesia. The designation of abnormal movements as either drug-related or intrinsically related to the schizophrenic illness on the basis of their characteristics is problematic (Owens, 1985; Barnes, 1988).

Videotape assessment

The use of videorecordings to assess patients with tardive dyskinesia would seem to have several practical advantages, not least being their availability for reappraisal at any convenient time. Videotapes are particularly useful for training raters and establishing some degree of inter-rater agreement on a particular scale before starting a research study. In treatment trials or follow-up studies where serial videotape recordings have been made of patients, the tapes may be shown to raters in random order so that they remain blind to the timing of the assessments.

A further methodological advantage is that all patients included in a study can be recorded in a standard fashion, engaged in the same activity (Fann *et al.*, 1977; Barnes and Trauer, 1982). Videotape recordings also allow close and prolonged observation of a patient that might be intrusive with a clinical observer, although some patients may be self-conscious and anxious in the presence of the camera which could affect their abnormal movements. While in theory, subtle abnormal movements may be more easily observed by a rater viewing a monitor screen than during a clinical examination (Asnis *et al.*, 1977), this will depend upon the quality and length of the recording, with fine movements perhaps only detectable in those body sites selected for close-up.

Two scales have been specifically designed for repeated evaluation, using standard videotape examination procedures: the Sct. Hans Rating Scale for Extrapyramidal Syndromes (see below) and the Tardive Dyskinesia Videotape Rating Scale (Barnes and Trauer, 1982). For both scales and associated videorecording examinations; satisfactory inter-rater reliability has been demonstrated (Gerlach and Korsgaard, 1983; Firth and Ardern, 1985; Fisk and York, 1987).

The various methods used to assess tardive dyskinesia may be loosely classified into those employing instrumentation, such as electromyography, ultrasound or digital image processing techniques, those using frequency counts of movements, and multi-item scales (Kane *et al.*, 1992). Multi-item scales are the most widely used method, and the most popular of these are described here.

Abnormal Involuntary Movement Scale (AIMS)
(Guy, 1976)

This scale is intended to assess the severity of abnormal involuntary movements in three general body regions: facial and oral movements are rated on four separate items; extremity movements on two separate items and trunk movement on one item. Each item is rated on a five-point scale (0-4) with instructions to rate the highest severity observed and to score movements that occur upon activation one less than those observed to occur spontaneously. The instrument also includes a global rating of severity, a rating of incapacitation due to abnormal movements and an item that assesses the patient's awareness of abnormal movements (each on a five-point scale). In addition, there are two items covering the patient's dental status. A standard examination procedure for the AIMS has been described.

Reliability and validity
Satisfactory levels of inter-rater have been demonstrated for the AIMS in several studies (Chien et al., 1977; Smith et al., 1979a,b; Whall et al., 1983; Lane et al., 1985). However, when Bergen et al. (1984) used the AIMS in an attempt to quantify the spontaneous fluctuations in tardive dyskinesia in a small group of patients, they found that within-rater variability dominated within-patient variability. They pointed out that to assess the change in tardive dyskinesia genuinely attributable to a therapeutic intervention or the passage of time, one would need to have information on the intra-rater and intra-patient variability in the condition.

In their prevalence studies of tardive dyskinesia using this scale, Smith et al. (1979a,b) found satisfactory inter-rater and test-retest reliability using the Pearson r correlation coefficient. However, they concluded that consistent bias may occur even with trained raters. Thus, they cautioned against using AIMS raters interchangeably in longitudinal assessments. Lane et al. (1985) examined inter-rater reliability in a sample of patients with tardive dyskinesia, using two experienced psychiatrists familiar with the AIMS and two residents with little previous exposure to patients with movement disorder. Analysis of the data revealed that the experienced raters obtained higher levels of agreement than the residents, and their scores were more consistent over time. These investigators calculated inter-rater reliability using both the Pearson r and the intraclass correlation coefficient recommended by Bartko and Carpenter (1976), on the suspicion that the former statistic provided an overestimate of the level of agreement. However, the correlations obtained by the two methods were very similar, and both showed high levels of agreement. The authors attributed these results, at least in part, to the conventions that they had developed for scoring the AIMS. These put forward additional criteria for rating severity on the dimensions of quality, frequency and amplitude, and also included guidelines for distinguishing between jaw and lip movement.

Utility
The AIMS scale ratings are based upon a standard examination procedure, appropriate for routine clinical evaluation of the condition. Clinicians of various disciplines may be easily trained to conduct and score the AIMS examination, which in routine clinical practice can be completed within 5-10 min (Germer et al., 1984; Munetz and Schulz, 1986). A Japanese version of the AIMS is available, for which inter-rater and test-retest reliability has been established (Itoh et al., 1977).

Two scoring conventions and guidelines for rating on the AIMS have been proposed (Lane *et al.*, 1985; Munetz and Benjamin, 1988), and these overlap on some points, but differ in other respects. For example, Munetz and Benjamin (1988) suggest that all hyperkinetic movements are rated regardless of presumed aetiology, so that the dyskinesia of Huntington's disease and Tourette's syndrome would be rated, while Lane *et al.* (1985) state that only movements of tardive dyskinesia should be rated, and specify that movements due to Huntington's disease, tics and tremors are excluded. Further, the original AIMS examination incorporated simple provocation tests, such as asking the patient to tap the tip of each finger in turn with the thumb. Any resultant "activated" movements that are observed are arbitrarily scored one less than those occurring spontaneously. Scores for both types of movement are added together for each body site rating. Potentially useful information is thus irretrievably buried within the total score (Barnes and Trauer, 1982). Munetz and Benjamin propose that a point is not subtracted from the score for movements seen only on activation. Their instruction is that the score should be determined "by considering the composite amplitude and frequency of movements that are qualitatively consistent with tardive dyskinesia". Lane and colleagues also suggest that movements occurring on activation are scored the same as spontaneous movements, except in the upper limbs, where finger movements occurring "in the passive hand in parallel with elicitation are scored one lower than finger movements not in parallel with elicitation".

Simpson Rating Scale for Tardive Dyskinesia
(Simpson et al. 1979)

This scale, developed by Simpson (1979) and sometimes referred to as the Rockland scale, provides 34 specific items rated on a six point scale (1 = absent to 6 = very severe). The items are clustered in five body regions: face; neck and trunk; upper extremities; lower extremities; and entire body. The scale also allows for additional items to be written in and rated. Several items included in the scale are not specific to tardive dyskinesia, for example, facial tics; pill-rolling movements; restless legs; akathisia. Definitions are provided for each item.

Reliability and validity
Reliability for a multi-item scale such as the Simpson scale is very variable on an item by item basis, but reliability is quite good for the global judgement item, which was added to the scale by other investigators. Kane *et al.* (unpublished data) tested the reliability of this scale with six raters examining 43 cases. Mean inter-rater reliability for the total score was 0.91 and 0.88 for the global severity rating. However, the figures for some of the other items, such as pouting and smacking and grimacing, were considerably lower, although limited variance was a factor. In contrast, using the smaller number of more global items of the AIMS tended to produce more consistent, higher reliability. This suggests that the detailed assessment of movements at a large number of body sites provided by lengthy multi-item

scales leads to more variance in ratings on specific items. A further issue relevant to achieving good inter-rater is the way investigators deal with the challenge of integrating reliability severity and frequency during the course of an examination. The instructions for the Simpson scale do not include substracting 1 from the rating if the movement is observed to occur only on activation.

Utility
The full-length version of the Simpson scale may be most useful in epidemiological and phenomenological investigations where considerable detail and refinement of assessment is desirable. It is perhaps not so well suited to assessing clinical change in the context of treatment trials. However, the abbreviated version is more appropriate in that context.

When analyzing the data from this scale, it is important to recognize that ratings on items such as pill-rolling movement or akathisia may contribute to the total score without necessarily being part of the syndrome of tardive dyskinesia.

Sct. Hans Rating Scale for Extrapyramidal Syndromes
(Gerlach, 1979; Gerlach and Korsgaard, 1983)

The Sct. Hans (also known as the Gerlach) Rating Scale for Extrapyramidal Syndromes distinguishes between hyperkinesia in the passive phase, when patients are sitting and relaxed, and movements observed in the active phase, when the patient is speaking or performing motor tasks such as writing or walking. The passive and active movement scores are added together for each of the body sites and the mean score calculated.

The scale was designed to be used for repeated evaluation, using videotape recordings. A standard video examination procedure is recommended, and the examination and recording take only 5-7 min (Korsgaard *et al.*, 1989). The scale covers parkinsonism, dystonia and akathisia, as well as tardive dyskinesia. When rating from a videotape there is a problem rating parkinsonian features such as rigidity and salivation, and the presence of these must be indicated by the examiner during the recording. This scale and the videorecording procedure have been successfully employed in a clinical multicenter study (Nordic Dyskinesia Study Group, 1986).

Rogers Motor Disorder Scale
(Rogers, 1985)

This scale was designed to rate movement disorder in schizophrenic patients, avoiding assumptions about a psychiatric or neurological aetiology. However, it was acknowledged that some of the movements rated would be regarded as drug-induced while others were more typical of the classical catatonic features of schizophrenia. More recently, the scale has been used in a large sample of individuals with mental handicap (Rogers *et al.*, 1991).

The original scale has been modified (Lund *et al.*, 1990). The revised version of the Rogers Motor Disorder Scale comprises 36 items, rating the severity of each abnormality on a three-point scale: absent (0), definitely present (1) and marked or pervasive (2). The items are grouped under headings such as disturbance of posture, tone, purposive movement and speech. The abnormalities considered to represent drug-induced parkinsonian and dyskinetic phenomena are identified, and the authors of the scale claim that the exclusion of these after the scale has been completed allows for the isolation of presumptive catatonic features.

The Dyskinesia Identification System – Coldwater (DIS-Co) The Dyskinesia Identification System: Condensed User Scale (DISCUS)
(Sprague et al., 1984a,b)

The DIS-Co was specifically developed for the assessment of mentally-retarded individuals. It has 34 items, derived from data collected on 519 "institutionalized mentally-retarded residents", 250 of whom had never received antipsychotic medication (Sprague *et al.*, 1984a). Subsequently, these investigators used the scale in a clinical study comparing three randomly-assigned treatment groups: a group receiving gradual reduction of their antipsychotic medication; a group receiving antipsychotic drugs without reduction; and a group who had not received antipsychotic drugs for at least 5 years. Sprague *et al.* (1984b) then revised the DIS-Co, based on the data collected in these studies. They developed a method for selecting items for the rating scale based on six qualities, including inter-rater reliability, stability and relationship with medication. The resulting 15-item scale, the DISCUS, has been used in training clinicians to assess tardive dyskinesia (Kalachnik *et al.*, 1988).

Reliability and validity
The inter-rater reliability, test-retest reliability and means and standard deviations for the items of the DISCUS scale items have been provided, based on 400 individuals with developmental disability (Sprague *et al.*, 1989).

Comparative Utility

The multi-item scales have proved the most popular instruments for the assessment of tardive dyskinesia, and the AIMS is the most widely used. Other scales commonly used include the Simpson scale (see above) and the Chouinard Extrapyramidal Rating Scale (Chouinard *et al.*, 1980). The main advantage of these scales is that they provide a comprehensive rating of the abnormal involuntary movements at the various body sites. Further, some of the scales have a recommended examination procedure, so their administration is standardized to some extent. However, for some AIMS there is more than one version of the guidelines for conducting the assessment examination (Lane *et al.*, 1985; Munetz and Benjamin, 1988).

Some authors have considered these scales be particularly suitable for screening populations for tardive dyskinesia (Munetz and Schulz, 1986; Ahrens *et al.*, 1988), on the basis that they are relatively inexpensive and unobtrusive, take only a short time to administer and may be applied to almost all patients.

The multi-item rating scales have not been designed as diagnostic instruments, although they usefully quantify the motor phenomena present and thereby contribute to the diagnostic process. In this context, it is useful for threshold scores to be employed in order to establish the minimum degree of motor abnormality necessary to qualify as a "case". For example, Schooler and Kane (1982) suggested that to warrant a diagnosis of tardive dyskinesia, the abnormal, involuntary movements should be rated as at least "moderate" severity on the AIMS in one or more body areas, or at least "mild" severity at two or more body sites. However, such criteria are essentially arbitrary and principally relevant to generating comparable research data rather than clinical diagnosis.

A further disadvantage is that the relatively simple, quantitative measures of frequency, amplitude or duration of movement used in most multi-item rating scales may allow for abnormal movements to be rated that are not specific to tardive dyskinesia. This is particularly a problem in the assessment of tardive dyskinesia of the extremities, as the scales may fail to differentiate between the choreiform, or choreo-athetoid dyskinesia considered characteristic of the condition, and other abnormal involuntary trunk and limb movements that may be present in chronic psychiatric patients. These include the movements associated with tardive dystonia and chronic akathisia as well as spontaneous motor disturbance related to psychotic illness. Although such movements are not part of the tardive dyskinesia syndrome, and may be pathophysiologically distinct, they may still be rated and thus contribute to the total scale score which may then be taken as a measure of the severity of tardive dyskinesia.

Conclusion

We have attempted to provide a brief discussion of several instruments available for the assessment of drug-induced movement disorders. The choice of instrument(s) will be influenced by the needs of the particular clinical application or research trial. Clearly, these instruments are only as good as the training and rigour surrounding their application, and clinicians as well as investigators must be sensitive to their inherent limitations.

Given the spectrum of abnormal movement disorders associated with antipsychotic drug treatment, their diagnosis and assessment remains an important challenge. These adverse effects are important because of their potential to produce subjective distress and to interfere with optimum psychosocial and vocational adjustment.

Their accurate assessment is essential not only in facilitating appropriate clinical management, but also in enabling clinicians and investigators to carry out relative benefit to risk evaluations of new pharmacological agents (or combinations of medications). In addition, the heterogeneity of the movement disorders themselves, as well as variations in patient vulnerability may provide important clues not only to the relevant pathophysiology, but also to mechanisms of drug action and the neurobiology of psychoses.

References

Addonzio, G. and Alexopoulos, G.S. (1988). Drug-induced dystonia in young and elderly patients. *American Journal of Psychiatry,* **145**, 869-871.

Adler, L., Anfrist, B., Pseslow, E., Corwin, J., Malanski, R. and Rotrosen, J. (1986). A controlled assessment of propranolol in the treatment of neuroleptic-induced akathisia. *British Journal of Psychiatry,* **149**, 42-45.

Adler, L.A., Angrist, B., Reiter, S. and Rotrosen, J. (1989). Neuroleptic-induced akathisia: a review. *Psychopharmacology,* **97**, 1-11.

Ahrens, T.N., Sramek, J.J., Herrera, J.M., Jewett, C.M. and Alcorn, V.E. (1988). Pharmacy-based screening program for tardive dyskinesia. *Drug Intelligence and Clinical Pharmacology,* **22**, 205-208.

Asnis, G.M., Leopold, M.A., Buvoisin, R.C. *et al.* (1977). A survey of tardive dyskinesia in psychiatric outpatients. *American Journal of Psychiatry,* **134**, 1367-1370.

Ayd, F. (1961). A survey of drug-induced extrapyramidal reactions. *Journal of the American Medical Association,* **175**, 1054-1060.

Barnes, T.R.E. (1987). The present status of tardive dyskinesia and akathisia in the treatment of schizophrenia. *Psychiatric Developments,* **5**, 301-319.

Barnes, T.R.E. (1988). Tardive dyskinesia: risk factors, pathophysiology and treatment. *In* "Recent Advances in Clinical Psychiatry" Vol. 6. (Ed. K. Granville-Grossman), pp. 185-207. Churchill Livingstone, London.

Barnes, T.R.E., (1989). A rating scale for drug-induced akathisia. *British Journal of Psychiatry,* **154**, 672-676.

Barnes, T.R.E. (1990). Movement disorder associated with antipsychotic drugs: the tardive syndromes. *International Review of Psychiatry,* **2**, 355-366.

Barnes, T.R.E. and Braude, W.M. (1985). Akathisia variants and tardive dyskinesia. *Archives of General Psychiatry,* **42**, 874-878.

Barnes, T.R.E. and Trauer, T. (1982). Reliability and validity of a tardive dyskinesia videotape rating technique. *British Journal of Psychiatry,* **140**, 508-515.

Bartels, M., Heide, K., Mann, K. and Schied, H.W. (1987). Treatment of akathisia with lorazepam. An open clinical trial. *Pharmacopsychiatry,* **20**, 51-53.

Bartko, J., Carpenter, W. (1976). On the methods and theory of reliability. *Journal of Nervous and Mental Disease,* **163**, 307-317.

Bergen, J.A., Griffiths, D.A., Rey, J.M. *et al.* (1984). Tardive dyskinesia: fluctuating patient or fluctuating rater. *British Journal of Psychiatry,* **144**, 498-502.

Blom, S. and Ekbom, K.A. (1961). Comparison between akathisia developing on treatment with phenothiazine derivatives and the restless legs syndrome. *Acta Medica Scandinavica,* **170**, 689-694.

Blowers A.J., Borison, R.L., Blowers, C.M. *et al.* (1981). Abnormal involuntary movements in the elderly. *British Journal of Psychiatry,* **139**, 363-364.

Braude, W.M., Barnes, T.R.E. and Gore, S.M. (1983). Clinical characteristics of akathisia:

a systematic investigation of acute psychiatric inpatient admissions. *British Journal of Psychiatry*, **143**, 139-150.

Burke, R.E., Fahn, S., Jankovic, J. *et al.* (1982). Tardive dystonia: late-onset and persistent dystonia caused by antipsychotic drugs. *Neurology*, **32**, 1335-1346.

Burke, R.E., Fahn, S., Marsden, C.D. *et al.* (1985). Validity and reliability of a rating scale for the primary torsion dystonias. *Neurology*, **35**, 73-77.

Burke, R.E., Kang, U.J., Jankovic, J., Miller, L.G. and Fahn, S. (1989). Tardive akathisia: an analysis of clinical features and response to open therapeutic trials. *Movement Disorders*, 1-19.

Casey, D.E. and Hansen, T.E. (1984). Spontaneous dyskinesias. *In* "Neuropsychiatric Movement Disorders" (Eds D.V. Jeste and R.J. Wyatt), pp. 68-95. American Psychiatric Press, Washington DC.

Casey, D.E., Gerlach, J., Magelund, G. *et al.* (1980). r-acetylenic GABA in tardive dyskinesia. *Archives of General Psychiatry*, **37**, 1376-1379.

Chien, C., Jung, K., Ross-Townsend, A. *et al.* (1977). The measurement of persistent dyskinesia by piezoelectric recording and clinical rating scales. *Psychopharmacology Bulletin*, **13**, 34-36.

Chouinard, G., Ross-Chouinard, A., Annable, L. and Jones, B.D. (1980). Extrapyramidal rating scale. *Canadian Journal of Neurological Science*, **7**, 233.

Dufresne, R.L. and Wagner, R.L. (1988). Antipsychotic-withdrawal akathisia versus antipsychotic-induced akathisia: further evidence for the existence of tardive akathisia. *Journal of Clinical Psychiatry*, **49**, 435-438.

Fahn, S. (1987). Systemic therapy of dystonia. *Canadian Journal of Neurological Science*, **14**, 528-532.

Fann, W.E., Stafford, J.E., Malone, R.L., *et al.* (1977). Clinical research techniques in tardive dyskinesia. *American Journal of Psychiatry*, **134**, 759-762.

Firth, W.R. and Ardern, M.H. (1985). Measuring abnormal movements in tardive dyskinesia: a pilot study. *British Journal of Psychiatry*, **147**, 723-726.

Fisk, G.G. and York, S.M. (1987). The effect of sodium valproate on tardive dyskinesia – revisited. *British Journal of Psychiatry*, **150**, 542-546.

Fleischhaker, W.W., Bengmann, K.J., Perovich, R., Pestreich, L.K., Borenstein, M., Lieberman, J.A. and Kane, J.M. (1989). The Hillside akathisia scale: a new rating instrument for neuroleptic-induced akathisia, parkinsonism and hyperkinesia. *Psychopharmacology Bulletin*, **25**, 222-226.

Fleischhaker, W.W., Miller, C.H., Schett, P., Barnes, C., Ehrmann, H. (1991). The Hillside Akathisia Scale: a reliability comparison of the English and German versions. *Psychopharmacology*, **105**, 141-144.

Friis, T., Christensen, T.R. and Gerlach, J. (1982). Sodium valproate and biperiden in neuroleptic-induced akathisia, parkinsonism and hyperkinesia. *Acta Psychiatrica Scandinavica*, **67**, 178-187.

Gardos, G. and Cole, J.O. (1980). Problems in the assessment of tardive dyskinesia. *In* "Tardive Dyskinesia: research and treatment". (Eds W.E. Fahn., R.C. Smith., J.M. Davis and E.F. Domino), pp. 201-214. Spectrum Publications, New York.

Gerlach, J. (179). Tardive dyskinesia. *Danish Medical Bulletin*, **26**, 209-245.

Gerlach, J. and Korsgaard, S. (1983). Classification of abnormal involuntary movements in psychiatric patients. *Neuropsychiatry Clinic*, **2**, 201-208.

Germer, C.K., Seraydarian, L. and McBrearty, J.F. (1984). Training hospital clinicians to diagnose tardive dyskinesia. *Hospital and Community Psychiatry*, **35**, 769-770.

Gibb, W.R.G. and Lees, A.J. (1986). The clinical phenomenon of akathisia. *Journal of Neurology, Neurosurgery and Psychiatry,* **49**, 861-866.

Guy, W. (1976). "ECDEU Assessment Manual for Psychopharmacology" revised edition. Washington DC, US Department of Health, Education and Welfare. Publication (ADM) 76-338, 1976, pp. 534-537.

Hershey, L.A., Gift, T. and Rivera-Calimlin, L. (1982). Not Parkinson's disease. *Lancet,* **2**, 49.

Inada, T., Yagi, G., Kamijima, K. *et al.* (1990). A statistical trial of subclassification for tardive dyskinesia. *Acta Psychiatrica Scandinavica,* **82**, 404-407.

Itoh, H., Yagi, G., Ogita, K., Ohtuka, N., Sakurai, S., Suzuki, T., Tashiro, I., Kaizawa, S., Kamijima, K., Koga, Y., Miura, S. (1977). The assessment of tardive dyskinesia by the AIMS (Japanese version). *Annual Report of Pharmacopsychiatry Research Foundation,* **39**, 1172-177.

Kalchnik, J.E., Sprague, R.L. and Slaw, K.M. (1988). Training clinical personnel to assess for tardive dyskinesia. *Progress in Neuropsychopharmacology, Biology and Psychiatry,* **12**, 749-762.

Kane, J.M., Weinhold, P., Kinon, B., Wegner, J. and Leader, M. (1982). Prevalence of abnormal involuntary movements ("spontaneous dyskinesias") in the normal elderly. *Psychopharmacology,* **77**, 105-108.

Kane, J.M., Rifkin, A., Woerner, M., Reardon, G., Sarantakos, S., Schiebel, D. and Ramos-Lorenzi, J. (1983). Low-dose neuroleptic treatment of outpatient schizophrenics: I. Preliminary results for relapse rates. *Archives of General Psychiatry,* **40**, 893-896.

Kane, J.M., Jeste, D.V., Barnes, T.R.E. *et al.* (1992). Assessment of tardive dyskinesia. *In* "Tardive Dyskinesia: a Task Force Report of the American Psychiatric Association". pp. 35-39. American Psychiatric Association, Washington.

Korsgaard, S., Gerlach, J., Noring, U. *et al.* (1989). Reliability and validity of the Sct. Hans rating scale for extrapyramidal syndromes. Unpublished manuscript.

Lane, R.D., Glazer, W.M., Hansen, T.E., Berman, W.H. and Kramer, S.I. (1985). Assessment of tardive dyskinesia using the abnormal involuntary movements scale. *Journal of Nervous and Mental Disease.* **173**, 353-357.

Lund, C.E., Mortimer, A.M., Rogers, D. and McKenna, P.J. (1991). Motor, volitional and behavioural disorders in schizophrenia. I: Assessment using the modified Rogers scale. *British Journal of Psychiatry,* in press.

Marsden, C.D., Tarsy, D. and Baldessarini, R.J. (1975). Spontaneous and drug-induced movement disorders in psychotic patient. *In* "Psychiatric Aspects of Neurological Disease". (Eds D.F. Benson and D. Blumer). pp. 219-266. Grune and Stratton, New York.

Miller, C.H., Fleischhaker, W.W., Ehrmann, J., Kane, J.M. (1990). Treatment of neuroleptic-induced akathisia with the 5-HT2 antagonist ritanserin. *Psychopharmacology Bulletin,* **26**, 373-376.

Mindham, R.H.S. (1976). Assessment of drug-induced extrapyramidal reactions and of drugs given for their control. *British Journal of Clinical Pharmacology,* Suppl. 395-400.

Munetz, M. and Benjamin, S. (1988). How to examine patients using the abnormal involuntary movement scale. *Hospital and Community Psychiatry,* **39**, 1172-1177.

Munetz, M.R. and Schulz, S.C. (1986). Screening for tardive dyskinesia. *Journal of Clinical Psychiatry,* **47**, 75-77.

Nordic Dyskinesia Study Group, (1986). Effect of different neuroleptics in tardive dyskinesia and parkinsonism. A video-controlled multicenter study with chlorprothixene, perphenazine, haloperidol and haloperidol + biperiden. *Psychopharmacology,*

90, 423-429.

Owens, D.G.C. (1985). Involuntary disorders of movement in chronic schizophrenia – The role of the illness and its treatment. *In* "Dyskinesia – Research and Treatment". (Eds D.E. Casey., A.V. Christensen.and J. Gerlach), pp. 79-87. Springer-Verlag, Berlin.

Richardson, M.A., Craig, T.J. and Branchey, M.H. (1982). Intra-patient variability in the measurement of tardive dyskinesia. *Psychopharmacology, 76*, 269-227.

Rifkin, A., Quitkin, F., Kane, J.M., Struve, F. and Klein, M. D.F. (1978). Are prophylactic antiparkinsonian drugs necessary? A controlled study of procyclidine withdrawal. *Archives of General Psychiatry, 35*, 483-489.

Rogers, D. (1985). The motor disorders of severe psychiatric illness: a conflict of paradigms. *British Journal of Psychiatry, 147*, 221-232.

Rogers, D., Karki, C., Bartlett, C. *et al.* (1991). The motor disorders of mental handicap: an overlap with the motor disorders of severe psychiatric illness. *British Journal of Psychiatry, 158*, 97-102.

Rupniak, N.M.J., Jenner, P. and Marsden, C.D. (1986). Acute dystonia induced by neuroleptic drugs. *Psychopharmacology, 88*, 403-419.

Schooler, N.R. and Kane, J.M. (1982). Research diagnosis for tardive dyskinesia (RD-TD). *Archives of General Psychiatry, 39*, 486-487.

Schwab, R.S. and England, A.C. Jr. (1968). Parkinson symptoms due to various specific causes. *In* "Handbook of Clinical Neurology, Diseases of the Basal Ganglia". Vol. 6. (Eds P.J. Vinken and G.W. Bruyn), pp. 227-247. North Holland, Amsterdam.

Sethi, K.D., Hess, D.C. and Harp, R.J. (1990). Prevalence of dystonia in veterans on chronic antipsychotic therapy. *Movement Disorders, 5*, 319-321.

Simpson, G.M. and Angus, J.W.S. (1970). A rating scale for extrapyramidal side-effects. *Acta Psychiatrica Scandinavica, 212*, (Suppl 44) 11-19.

Simpson, G.M., Lee, J.H., Zoubok, B., Cole, J.O. and Gardos, G. (1979). A rating scale for tardive dyskinesia. *Psychopharmacology, 64*, 171-179.

Smith, J.M., Kucharski, L.T., Oswald, W.T. and Waterman, L.J. (1979a). A systematic investigation of tardive dyskinesia in schizophrenic inpatients. *American Journal of Psychiatry, 136*, 918-922.

Smith, J.M., Kucharski, L.T., Eblen, C. *et al.* (1979b). An assessment of tardive dyskinesia in schizophrenic outpatients. *Psychopharmacology, 64*, 99-104.

Sprague, R.L., Kalachnik, J.E., Breuning, S.E., Davis, V.J., Ullman, R.K., Cullari, S., Davidson, N.A., Ferguson, D.G. and Hoffner, B.A. (1984a). The dyskinesia identification sysiem – coldwater DIS-CO: a tardive dyskinesia rating scale for the developmentally disabled. *Psychopharmacology Bulletin, 20*, 328-338.

Sprague, R.L., White, D.M., Ullman, R. and Kalachnik, J.E. (1984b). Methods for selecting items in a tardive dyskinesia rating scale. *Psychopharmacology Bulletin, 20*, 339-345.

Sprague, R.L., Kalachnik, J.E. and Shaw, M. (1989). Psychometric properties of the Dyskinesia Identification System: Condensed User Scale (DISCUS). *Mental Retardation, 27*, 141-148.

Van Putten, T. and Marder, S.R. (1986). Toward a more reliable diagnosis of akathisia. *Archives of General Psychiatry, 43*, 1015-1016.

Van Putten, T. and Marder, S.R. (1987). Behavioural toxicity of antipsychotic drugs. *Journal of Clinical Psychiatry, 48*, (Suppl. 9) 13-19.

Walters, A.S. and Hening, A. (1989). Opioids a better treatment for acute than tardive akathisia: possible role for the endogenous opiate system in neuroleptic-induced akathisia. *Medical Hypotheses, 28*, 1-2.

Webster, D.D. (1968). Clinical analysis of the disability in Parkinson's disease. *Modern Treatments,* **5**, 257-282.

Weiden, P.J., Mann, J.J., Haas, G., Mattson, M. and Frances, A. (1987). Clinical non-recognition of neuroleptic-induced movement disorders: a cautionary study. *American Journal of Psychiatry,* **144**, 1148-1153.

Weiner, W.J. and Luby, E.D. (1983). Persistent akathisia following neuroleptic withdrawal. *Annals of Neurology,* **13**, 466-467.

Whall, A.L., Engle, V., Edwards, A., Bodel, L. and Haberland, C. (1983). Development of a screening progamme for tardive dyskinesia: feasibility issues. *Nursing Research,* **32**, 151-156.

Woerner, M.G., Kane, J.M., Lieberman, J.A. *et al.* (1991). The prevalence of tardive dyskinesia. *Journal of Clinical Psychopharmacology,* **11**, 34-42.

Yassa, R., Nair, V. and Dimitry, R. (1986). Prevalence of tardive dystonia. *Acta Psychiatrica Scandinavica,* **73**, 629-633.

14. The Assessment of Aggression and Potential for Violence

Til Wykes, Richard Whittington and Robert Sharrock

Aggressive behaviour represents a considerable problem for psychiatric services. Apart from the obvious effects on the victims and the immediate management problems it poses, violence also complicates the course of treatment. It may lead to restrictive interventions, lengthen inpatient treatment and will make transfer to the community more difficult.

Unfortunately, over the past 10 years there has been evidence of a significant increase in violence by psychiatric patients which may be following the trends observed in society, e.g. that the incidence of serious crimes such as homicide increased by 30% and woundings and assaults nearly doubled between 1974 and 1984 (Walmsley, 1986). Within hospitals in the United Kingdom several studies have provided evidence of substantial increases in violent incidents. The rates of increase vary from 240% over 15 months in a high dependency psychiatric ward (James *et al.*, 1990) to 47% in a survey of health authorities (Rogers and Salvage, 1988). Similar variability has been found in America. The rates vary from a 316% increase in assaults on staff between 1975 and 1980 in a private psychiatric hospital (Adler *et al.*, 1983) to a 100% increase in injurious patient assaults on nurses over a 3-year period at a Los Angeles psychiatric hospital (Poster and Ryan, 1989). All these studies are on small samples over relatively short periods of time, the only study which has reported a large number of incidents over a significant period of time is Noble and Rodger's (1990) report on the Bethlem Royal and Maudsley Hospital Violent Incident Register. This shows that the number of violent incidents in 1987 was treble that in 1976.

Several reasons have been posited to account for the increase in violent incidents in hospitals. For instance the emphasis on community care may have affected the inpatient population that remains so that there is a higher proportion of seriously ill patients than before because the less ill have been discharged (Adler *et al.*, 1983; Haller and Deluty, 1988; Noble and Rodger, 1989). The population may also be less stable with more frequent re-admissions.

Most of the violence reported in hospitals is not physically severe. Eighty-five per cent of incidents surveyed by Cooper *et al.* (1983) and 69% of assaults in Convey's (1986) study produced little injury but as Conn and Lion (1983) point out the victims of this violence almost unanimously agreed that the emotional impact of an incident far exceeds the physical impact.

It is not possible to conclude that violence within hospitals is less severe than that in the community because comparisons are hindered by the non-reporting of minor incidents in the community. The evidence we do possess suggests that there are differences between cultures. American studies report higher levels in psychotic patients than those studies based in Europe and mirror differences in reported violence in the two communities.

All these data emphasize the urgency for the development of assessment procedures which will enable clinicians both to describe incidents and to predict who is likely to commit such acts and at what times. No satisfactory epidemiological evidence exists on the association between violence and psychosis but most reports indicate that patients with a diagnosis of schizophrenia present either the same but more often a higher risk than those without such illnesses and also higher than patients with other diagnoses (Fottrell, 1980; Armond, 1982; Aiken, 1984; Pearson *et al.*, 1986). It is therefore particularly important to investigate violence and aggression amongst this group.

Because of all the difficulties in the measurement and definition of violence (discussed below) the focus of this chapter will mainly be the assessment and prediction of violence among inpatients but reference will be made to assessment in the community where it is appropriate. First, we will outline the problems in the area, then we will describe factors which relate to aggression or its prediction in psychotic patients. Finally, we describe some scales and suggest a series of measures which will be of use in assessing violence and its prediction in psychotic patients.

Difficulties in measurement

Although there is evidence of increases in violence and that patients with psychoses are over-represented in the group of violent patients, the research on the relationship between psychosis and violence has been impaired by a lack of agreed measures and definitions. There are three major problems:

First, there is a lack of agreement on what constitutes violence. Even if violence is studied within a hospital setting there is still confusion. For instance, some studies include only assaults on staff, whereas others include assaults on patients (e.g. Convit *et al.*, 1988*b*) and visitors, as well as the destruction of property (e.g. Noble and Rodgers, 1990) and even self-harm (e.g. Janofsky *et al.*, 1988). Other researchers do not even provide a guide to what areas they did include (e.g. Palmstierna *et al.*, 1989). This limits the generalizability of much of the data.

Secondly, some studies include verbal abuse and threats (e.g. Kay *et al.*, 1988*a*), whilst others use physical contact as a criterion (e.g. Convit *et al.*, 1988*a*). Again, others are not explicit either way (e.g. Convit *et al.*, 1988*a*).

Thirdly, the way in which the aggressive or violent event has been notified is important because of the problem of under-reporting. Lion *et al.* (1981) compared officially reported incidents with those mentioned in the daily ward reports completed every 24 hours by staff on the ward and found that five times as many assaults occurred as were officially reported. Some researchers have side-stepped this problem by focusing on more physically serious incidents which, it is claimed

(Haller and Deluty, 1988) are more validly reported, or on repeatedly assaultive patients (Convit *et al.*, 1990). Still others have changed the phenomenon under study from the poorly-reported violent incident to the reporting of staff injury (Carmel and Hunter, 1989).

The observed incidence of violence in psychosis is also related to the nature of the sample under investigation. Much recent research on violence and psychosis deals with patients whose behaviour has necessitated hospital admission, sometimes in secure conditions, and on such samples it is difficult to make general inferences about the relationship between psychosis and violence.

Patients are also observed over varying time periods ranging from a few days following admission to months or years in the community.

Such vagaries partly account for the range in estimates of the incidence of aggression in psychosis from 8% to 45% (Volavka and Krakowski, 1989). Nevertheless, there is some agreement that the risk of violence in schizophrenia is higher, if only slightly, than in other patient groups or the general population (Rabkin, 1979). Clearly, even if psychosis and aggression are independent, a proportion of psychotic patients will exhibit aggressive behaviour.

Aggression is often defined as the intention to hurt or gain advantage over others, without necessarily involving physical harm that is a defining feature of violence (e.g. Howell and Hollin, 1989). Tedeschi *et al.* (1974) recast the concept of aggression in terms of coercive power in which punishment, actual or threatened, is used to obtain certain ends. However, this definition also places emphasis on the motives for violence which in practice are difficult to assess. The additional assumption that actors "always behave in a manner calculated to instrumentally attain planned outcomes" (Tedeschi *et al.* 1974, p. 549) seems dubious in the context of psychotic violence which is often notable for its random disregard of consequences.

It may be more sensible to define aggression in terms of its effects, such as behaviour which causes physical harm or psychological distress to others, so as to leave open for empirical research its association with internal states and causes. The distinction between covert feelings and thoughts of anger, and overt expressions of these states in the form of aggression or violence has been widely accepted, and emphasizes that aggression and violence are associated with, and may arise from internal states, both cognitive and emotional.

The Predictors of an Individual's Violence
Demographic factors
(i) *Gender* Women in psychiatric hospitals are likely to be more frequently aggressive than the female population. This may be because the effects of mental illness on violence, the feelings of paranoia or disinhibition, for instance, act equally on men and women. Alternatively, there is a view that violent women are more likely to become involved with the legal and psychiatric systems because aggression is viewed by society as "unfeminine".

Once in hospital there is little evidence that members of one sex are more frequently aggressive than others. Studies that have found differences have generally not controlled for the numbers of men and women in psychiatric hospitals. Larger studies which did control for hospital population (e.g. Hodgkinson et al., 1985; Blomhoff et al., 1990; Convit et al., 1990; James et al., 1990) found no significant differences between the sex ratios in violent and hospital populations overall. Although, Hodgkinson, McIvor and Phillips (1985) did find an effect for sex combined with age. Females aged under 20 years, 40-59 years and 70-79 years were involved in significantly more incidents than females of those ages in the hospital.

(ii) *Age*   The mean age of assaulting patients is little different from the hospital population but there is agreement that certain patients are more violent than others. In particular, patients in their twenties presented a higher risk. But violence occurs throughout the age range.

(iii) *Ethnicity*   Most studies have found no differences due to ethnicity or foreign birth. Noble and Rodger (1989) found a tendency for Afro-Caribbean patients to commit more serious assaults but these authors acknowledge that this group of patients are also provided with more restrictive forms of care and these differences may have affected the likelihood of violence.

History of Violence

One generalization derived from penal research is that the single best predictor of future aggression is previous aggression in relevant situations. This is mimicked both within hospitals and for psychiatric patients in the community. Monahan (1981, p.116) concluded that the higher rate of violent crime committed by former psychiatric patients is accounted for by those patients with a history of violence that preceded their hospitalization.

On the other hand, there are a small but important number of cases where aggression is causally related to psychosis, notably when patients act violently against others when in the active phase of illness, or more particularly, under the influence of delusions or paranoid ideas (Planansky and Johnston, 1977). Taylor (1985) surveyed psychotic offenders and found that 20% were actively driven to offend as a result of their symptoms.

Symptoms

Most reports indicate that patients with a diagnosis of schizophrenia present a higher risk than those with other diagnoses (Fottrell, 1980; Armond, 1982; Aiken, 1984; Pearson et al., 1986). This appears true even when the prevalence of this diagnosis within psychiatric hospitals has been taken into account (Cooper et al., 1983; Hodgkinson et al., 1985; Noble and Rodgers, 1989; James et al., 1990).

An examination of schizophrenic patients who have committed violent crimes revealed a very large proportion who had been psychotic at the time of the offence (Planansky and Johnston, 1977; Taylor, 1985). But Virkkunen (1974) reported that only a third of violent offences were committed during a psychotic episode. Differences between these studies may be explained by the lack of diagnostic criteria given by Virkkunen.

Nevertheless, it is thinking disturbance which is the best predictor of violence in ward settings over brief periods. Yesavage *et al.* (1981) showed that hallucinatory behaviour, conceptual disorganization and unusual thought content were significant predictors of violence over an 8 day period following admission. Tanke and Yesavage (1985) compared the symptom clusters measured on the Brief Psychiatric Rating Scale (BPRS) between high visibility patients who issued threats prior to the assault and low visibility patients who did not issue threats. Both groups of patients scored higher on thinking disorder and activation than the non-violent population. But only the high visibility patients were rated higher on the hostile-suspiciousness factor. In addition, the low visibility patients scored higher than both the high visibility and the non-violent population on the withdrawal-retardation factor. This study also found a further interesting result – those patients who were least predictable in their behaviour (i.e. issued no warnings) were the most predictable when BPRS scores were employed. That is, BPRS scores were most significantly related to violent behaviour only in those patients who did not provide any cues to their violence.

On the other hand, Palmstierna *et al.* (1989) showed that ratings of hostility and anxiety soon after admission predicted violence over an 8 or 28 day period. Their sample contained fewer schizophrenics than the other studies mentioned, so it is possible that distinct aspects of mental state have different predictive values depending on patient type. This study also did not analyze the circumstances of the violence, e.g. threats beforehand. Blomhoff *et al.* (1990) too found that levels of aggression were significantly lower for the violent group than for the non-violent group at referral and at admission. Aggression at referral and anxiety at admission correctly classified 78% of violent patients. Lowenstein *et al.* (1990) found that higher levels of thinking disturbance, hostile-suspiciousness and agitation-excitement measured by the BPRS on admission was significantly associated with violence during hospitalization.

Command hallucinations seem to play a minor role in the prediction of violence. They have never been identified as carrying a high degree of risk even if the behaviour is life threatening, or only minor assault (Hellerstein *et al.*, 1987).

Delusions, especially paranoid ones, are often cited as symptoms accompanying violent offences and some studies even claim this is the most important symptom in triggering violent behaviour among people with psychosis. People with delusions of misidentification, especially those which are well developed, have also been shown to be more likely to commit violent crimes against people although other features too must be taken into account (De Pauw and Szulecka, 1988). Many questions remain unanswered about the relationship between delusions and violence. For example, what is the nature of the triggering event, the relationship of delusions to other symptoms prior to violence and which details of the delusion would be important in prediction.

The type of violence also seems to be related to particular patterns of symptoms. Violence associated with paranoid delusions seems to be the sort that is well planned, directed at a significant individual in the patient's life and is often dangerous, whereas the violence associated with disorganized psychotic states is less focused and often less dangerous (Krakowski *et al.*, 1986).

Anti-psychotic medication tends to reduce the likelihood of violence, although the effects of medication are not always easy to disentangle from the effects of hospital admission. Removing a patient from his or her usual environment may be beneficial to the extent that violence and psychosis both reflect common causes such as social stresses (Taylor, 1985).

Volavka and Krakowski (1989) have hypothesized that there exists a sub-group of violent psychotic patients who are less responsive to neuroleptic medication and hospital admission. They suggest that there is a neurological basis for violence in this group and serotonergic mechanisms are involved. Although they argue that there is a need for more research to examine the complex interactions between environmental and neurological determinants of violence in psychosis.

Setting Conditions

The setting conditions include the physical location, type of ward, time of incident, atmosphere on the ward, etc. There is no agreement about the place where incidents occur. In some studies many occurred in common areas such as the dining room (Cooper *et al.*, 1983; Coldwell and Naismaith, 1990) whereas other studies found that the majority of incidents were in the dormitory (Drinkwater, 1982). Fottrell (1980) found that incidents mainly occurred on acute admission wards, drug dependency units and intensive treatment wards. In Hodgkinson *et al.* (1985) many incidents took place on the locked intensive care ward and most admission wards. There were low rates of incidents on the long-stay and psychogeriatric wards, and hardly any in the therapeutic community and alcohol/drug dependency wards.

The ward atmosphere has been thought to contribute to levels of violence although the specific type of atmosphere (controlling vs democracy) has not been shown to be related unequivocally to increases or otherwise of violence. James *et al.* (1990) found that when the proportion of permanent nursing staff halved over 15 months the number of incidents increased by 240%. There was a positive correlation between violence and agency provision and a negative one with permanent staff provision. There was no relationship with admission rates, bed occupancy or changes in medical staffing. Katz and Kirkland (1990) tried to distinguish violent and peaceful wards by an anthropological approach.

Characteristics of peaceful wards included predictable regular meetings and activities, patient participation and good staff communication and clear staff roles. Potential violence was met with consistent procedures carried out by a staff team calmly. It was made clear that violence was not allowed and incidents were thoroughly discussed afterwards. The atmosphere on violence prone wards was characterized by uncertainty, fear and confusion. Staff were isolated from the psychiatrist and from the patients; meetings and activities were irregular, occasional and *ad hoc*. Diagnosis was the aim not the beginning of treatment.

Summary

Demographic characteristics do not seem to differentiate violent from non-violent populations of patients. The relationships, if any, are more complicated than current studies have investigated. Apart from these characteristics patients with psychotic illnesses will differ in their past history of violence, their social skills and their symptomatology and these do appear to be important features in predicting aggression. Patients with a history of violence prior to a diagnosis of psychosis have a higher risk. Patients who have deficient assertiveness skills and therefore appear under- or over-controlled may also provide a risk (Megargee, 1966) although this is disputed. Different symptomatology may also help to define subgroups who are more or less prone to violence. The prediction of violence requires the consideration of all these factors although their relative weights in the prediction equation are currently unknown.

The Assessment Procedures

What is aggression and the potential for violence? The measures described below fall into two categories. The first is concerned with rating observed aggression, usually in the form of behavioural rating scales. The second is concerned with the capacity or potential for aggression.

Rating Scales of Observed Aggression

In order for observer ratings to be accurate, the definitions of behaviour should be objective, clear and complete. Objectivity here is taken to mean that the definition should refer to observable events or behaviour. Clarity relates to the ease with which a definition can be communicated with other raters without a change in meaning; and completeness specifies the boundary conditions of what is or is not included in the definition. The assessment of inter-rater agreement or "reliability" is an important check that these criteria are satisfied. A final criterion is sensitivity, and refers to the ability to discriminate between different degrees of aggression. If the assessment is designed to measure change then sensitivity is a crucial and often overlooked characteristic of any rating scale.

The following description of assessment devices is not intended to provide an exhaustive summary. Rather it provides the reader with the advantages of various methods to facilitate the selection or derivation of a suitable recording method for their own purposes.

The Overt Aggression Scale (OAS)
(Yudofsky et al., 1986)

This scale was originally designed to assess the effect of propranolol on aggression. It is a simple staff rating scale of four types of aggression: verbal, physical, abuse of objects and self abuse. These four categories each contain four severity levels.

The scale also provides a list of interventions which could be employed. The total aggression score is derived by adding the subscores, with added weight given to more severe forms of aggression.

Reliability and validity
Most items had adequate inter-rater reliabilities in excess of 0.75, although some categories have rather fuzzy definitions and the standardization was carried out on very small samples. The validity coefficients are generally low and non-significant.

Utility
The meaning of the total sum is rather arbitrary as it requires summing the most aggressive behaviours with the nature of the staff interventions. These interventions will vary according to institutional policies as well as other factors.

The Modified Overt Aggression Scale (MOAS)
(Kay et al., 1988a)

This scale, as its name implies, is derived from the Overt Aggression Scale (Yudofsky et al., 1986). The MOAS was produced in order to overcome some of the limitations of the OAS, including lack of definitions for the categories and the exclusion of certain aggressive acts, such as suicide attempts and intimidation, as well as the arbitrariness of the total score. The MOAS was standardized on over 250 adult patients, 81% of whom were psychotic. Ratings of the most severe form of aggression within each of four categories were performed daily by psychiatrists, clinical psychologists or psychiatric social workers in co-operation with primary care staff. These were based on the "totality of information" including personal observations, ward records and conversations with staff. The categories of violence are: verbal aggression, aggression against property, autoaggression and physical aggression. In this scale the classes of aggression are better defined and more clearly form five-point ordinal scales.

Reliability and validity
Inter-rater reliability coefficients are reported only for the total score rather than within classes of aggression but they are generally high (Pearson's r: Inter-rater 0.85-0.94; Test-retest 0.72) but short term stability of score was only found in one subgroup.

Utility
The scale was shown to discriminate levels of aggression between settings, but its predictive validity in relation to non-hospital settings is unknown. Sensitivity could be increased by noting the frequency of behaviours within each category per unit of time.

The Staff Observation Aggression Scale (SOAS)
(Palmstierna and Wistedt, 1987)

The SOAS is a practical means of assessment designed for nursing staff to systematically record an aggressive incident when it arises. It aims to capture not only the aggressive behaviour itself, but also the provocation, if any, and the consequences and interventions that ensued.

Utility
Although the severity of aggression is measured in terms of its "means" (e.g. verbal, parts of the body, or weapons); "aims" (e.g. object, staff or patient); or result (e.g. damage to people or objects), there is insufficient detail in the coding of aggression so it is unclear whether the scale has sufficient precision to detect subtle change. Furthermore, it is not clear on what basis an aggressive event was recorded at all, although it is to be expected that the decision to report an incident will depend on factors other than the behaviour, for example, staff tolerance and availability of time. The scale has yet to be extensively standardized.

Scale for the Assessment of Aggressive and Agitated Behaviours (SAAB)
(Brizer et al., 1987)

The SAAB is another systematic means of recording aggressive events as and when they occur. Aggression is defined as "agitation, verbal assault, asault against the self ..., other ..., to property". The context of the incident in terms of setting, background agitation and the consequences of aggression are also recorded. Unsurprisingly, "agitation" proved a difficult concept to operationalize, as evidenced by its poor reliability. The scale is completed by professional staff and the study confirms that ward-based records are likely to under-report moderate or minor aggressive incidents.

Aggression Risk Profile
(Kay et al., 1988b)

This profile is based on a series of studies which aimed to characterize the aggressive patient. The predictive power was based on a study of 208 subjects which tested 39 variables. These were reduced to 19 which provided reasonable concurrent or predictive validity for violence measured on the MOAS. The items include a clinical profile which has measures of behaviour, e.g. motor excitement, agitation, delusions and hallucinations as well as measures of social skills, e.g. low tolerance to frustration, difficulty in delaying gratification, antisocial behaviour. The other dimensions are demographic characteristics, diagnosis (using DSM III criteria) and history of aggression. The final scale includes four anchored points for levels of severity.

Reliability and validity

The inter-rater concordance was significant for all items of the condensed scale (mean $r = 0.72$). Significant longitudinal reliability was obtained for all but the clinical profile, although some items making up the profile did achieve reasonable reliability. Interestingly, the contemporaneous covariates of aggression were not the same as the predictors. Different measures were also found for verbal, physical and total aggression. The most reliable predictors were younger age, shorter length of illness, hostility, depression, anger and difficulty in delaying gratification.

Utility

This sort of scale is likely to be useful in the future, but further testing in different settings with different sorts of raters is essential before it can be used to motivate prevention.

Self Report Measures

Self report measures have great appeal because of their apparent objectivity, ease of administration and simplicity of scoring. However, it is well known that responding to questionnaires is affected by a number of biases, including acquiescence and the tendency to respond in a socially acceptable manner. Further, in psychotic groups there is particular difficulty in ensuring that patients co-operate and fully comprehend the meaning of questions.

Although acquiescence can be minimized by careful item construction, there are greater difficulties with the effects of social desirability since aggression is widely seen as unacceptable and individuals may be particularly motivated to present in an acceptable way to expedite their discharge. This may explain Selby's (1984) counter-intuitive finding that prison inmates had lower ratings of anger using Novaco's (1975) inventory (see below) than non prison controls.

Faking assumes that the responder has correctly inferred the content of the item, and there is evidence that more direct measures such as the Buss-Durkee Inventory are easier to fake good and bad (depending on the motivation of the responder) than more obtuse measures such as the MMPI. The lesson for the clinician is to be aware both of the patient's motivations and the limitations of the questionnaire. Measures of social desirability, such as the Lie-Scale from the Eysenck Personality Questionnaire (1975) may also be administered to assess social presentation.

These difficulties may explain the poor predictive validity of questionnaire measures of the potential for violence. In a most comprehensive review and following their own extensive research, Edmunds and Kendrick (1980) concluded that there was no convincing demonstration of the value of paper and pencil tests in predicting actual aggression. They argued that to predict aggression an analysis of the individual's situation and provocations was required. Even when tests do seem to predict violence with some success this is often on the basis of *post-hoc* statistical procedures such as discriminant function analysis: the subsequent step, of validating the predictive equations thus derived against a separate sample, is usually notable by its absence. In spite of these limitations these scales are popular and so are briefly described below.

Buss-Durkee Hostility Inventory
(Buss and Durkee, 1957)

After defining sub-classes of hostility, the authors devised 105 items which was reduced to 75 following statistical analysis. Classes of hostility were: assault, indirect aggression (including temper tantrums and door slamming), irritability, negativism, resentment, suspicion and verbal hostility.

Reliability and validity
There was an effect of social desirability, but a small one: ratings of the social desirability of each item correlated approximately 0.3 with actual responding to each item, in contrast to much higher correlations in other research using this procedure (Edwards, 1954). Factor Analysis revealed two factors: an emotional-attitudinal component, including resentment and suspiciousness and a motor component including overt aggression and irritability. These factors map closely on to those derived from Kendrick and Edmunds' research, who found in males and from a number of inventories two overall dimensions from factor analysis: hostility and aggressiveness.

Utility
The Buss-Durkee is one of the most widely used questionnaires of hostility and aggression. It has reasonable correlations with other anger inventories and it has been shown to differentiate violent from non-violent prison populations. But, its predictive validity is poor or non-existent. The usefulness of this sort of scale in assessing violence among psychotic patients is currently unknown.

Novaco Anger Inventory
(Novaco, 1975)

In contrast to the approach of Buss and Durkee in identifying types of aggressive responsiveness, Novaco's approach has been to identify a set of situations that may evoke anger, including provocation, threats to self-esteem and frustration, and to measure how much subjective anger each evokes on a five-point scale. The scale focuses on covert hostility and the situations which elicit it rather than overt aggression.

Reliability and validity
One benefit of this simplifying approach is high levels of internal reliability – as high as 0.96 for a sample of university students. It correlates highly with a similar scale (Reaction Inventory: Evans and Strangeland, 1971), but weakly with the Buss-Durkee, showing it is measuring a distinct aspect of aggression.

Utility

There are, of course, limitations. First, evidence concerning predictive validity is lacking, although Selby (1984) did find large and statistically significant differences between violent and non-violent offenders. Second, it has not been standardized on psychotic patients or mentally abnormal offenders. Thirdly, the content validity of the scale depends on the degree of overlap between the situations tapped by the questionnaire and real life anger-arousing situations that are relevant to the respondent. Since the scale has been designed around the problems faced by university students, there is little reason to suppose it is directly relevant to psychiatrically ill patients. On the other hand, treatment studies using NAI show it to be sensitive to change (e.g. Hazaleus and Deffenbacher, 1986), so the scale may be useful in evaluating interventions, even if the translation of scores into an appraisal of the risk of violence is difficult.

In a recent paper Novaco (1991) reports that anger rated in annual surveys of the California State Hospitals is predictive of aggression in the following year, even when other factors, such as assaults in the year of the anger rating, depression psychotic symptoms and demographic factors are all controlled. There is therefore a need to adapt and develop further methods of measuring anger within the psychotic population.

The MMPI and Derivative Scales

It was the failure of MMPI indices of hostility to differentiate violent and non-violent offenders that has led to the development of Megargee's (1967) Overcontrolled-Hostility Scale and recently Blackburn's Assessment Schedules which are discussed here.

(i) Overcontrolled-Hostility Scale
(Megargee et al., 1967)

Megargee's concept of the overcontrolled personality attempted to explain how some people, with rigid defences against the expression of aggression, may react catastrophically to an apparently minor provocation. The theory is that aggressive motivation may summate in a manner similar to other drives such as hunger or thirst. No research convincingly demonstrates the increased risk of extreme assaultiveness in "over-controlled" individuals. Indeed, McGurk (1980) noted that 72% of prison officers emerged as over-controlled; and showed substantially less over-control in a group of murderers, directly at odds with Megargee's predictions.

(ii) Blackburn's Assessment Schedules
(Blackburn, 1968a,b, 1987)

Blackburn has conducted research into the personality of mentally abnormal offenders, using the SHAPS (Special Hospital Assessment of Personality and

Socialisation), a multi-trait questionnaire derived from the MMPI, the Buss-Durkee Inventory, and the Psychopathic Delinquency Scale. Factor analysis consistently reveals two major factors. The first is essentially one of hostility, which Blackburn refers to as Belligerence, which loads on impulsivity, aggression and negatively with the Lie Scale. The second factor is one of inhibition and social avoidance, referred to as Withdrawal, reflecting a dimension of control. The evidence concerning both internal and test-retest reliabilities is convincing, particularly for Belligerence, although the Withdrawal factor showed a high (-0.53) correlation with Eysenck's Lie Scale, suggesting that responses are being affected by dissimulation. It is the controlled patients, often with one previous offence of homicide against a family member, who seem to have a better prognosis on discharge (Black, 1987). Those with worse prognosis from special hospitals have previous convictions and show psychopathic traits such as impulsiveness and hostile attitudes to others (Black, *op. cit.*), aspects which are tapped by the B scale. Unfortunately, there is little objective evidence to date which bears upon the predictive validity of the SHAPS even though its primary use is in the evaluation and prediction within forensic and penal populations.

A Basic Clinical Guide to Assessment of Imminent Violence

There is a need for a range of assessments of different types as well as a range of possible outcome measures.

The outcome measures, incidents of violence, are fairly easy to record using the Modified Overt Aggression Scale (Kay *et al.,* 1988a), although this scale also needs to have information on the context of aggression. For example, was the aggression planned, was there provocation, was it a response to restrictions within the psychiatric ward? All these setting factors will enable an individual picture of violence to be developed.

The clinical assessment should include symptoms, especially delusions. Several assessments may be useful and overall symptom descriptions, e.g. BPRS as well as more detailed accounts of particular symptoms, e.g. the form and content of delusions. The person's support systems, ability to co-operate with treatment, violent ideation, and recent and past history of violence will all aid an assessment, particularly for imminent violence.

Information on the person's social skills, their ability to deal with frustration and their ability to communicate their needs would also add to the picture. These could also be carried out between, as well as within, a psychotic episode as a basis for intervention.

Conclusion

It is surprising that given the length of time in which this subject has interested the psychiatric professions there is no agreed method for delineating what a violent incident is or how it should be recorded. One problem has been to acknowledge the heterogeneity of aggression and violence between individuals, over contexts and over time. This is particularly true for people with psychotic illnesses whose potential for violence is also affected by their psychotic experiences and their reactions to them.

The main conclusion to be drawn from this review of the area is that the choice of assessment instruments depends on the questions that need to be answered. Comparisons of violence between populations and between settings require more global scales that are accurate in different settings. These new assessments also need to be developed to record aggression over particular time periods, e.g. violence within 10 days of admissions. The current scales all have their deficiencies so there is plenty of room to develop further scales or to incorporate the best aspects of each.

If the question is about individual cases or the building up of a catalogue of violent incidents then there is an emphasis on collecting more detailed information about the incidents themselves. This information would allow consideration of clusters of incidents in relation to individual characteristics such as symptoms, warning signals and social skills. This question of the specificity of violence within and across individuals should be the main research focus.

Many of the current assessments provide little detail of the setting and context factors involved in violent incidents for particular individuals. One convincing argument for detailing context is given by Hinde (1990) using an ethological approach. He emphasized the need to consider diverse motivations in the assessment of violence. For instance, some aggression may involve both aggressiveness and specific acquisitiveness (the motivation to acquire some object) whilst in other cases aggressiveness and assertiveness (motivation to enhance one's status) may be involved. Even if psychosis increases the propensity for violence, specific motivational prerequisites need to be appraised if the prediction of violence within an individual is to be improved.

The prediction of the likelihood of violence is an assessment that clinicians are expected to make on a daily basis in order to prescribe treatment. Within the confines of the Mental Health Act they are also asked to decide whether someone is a "danger to others." These decisions need to be motivated by research findings that use reliable methods of assessment and which produce useful clinical tools for the prediction of violence.

References

Adler, W.A., Kreeger, C. and Ziegler, P. (1983). Patient violence in a private psychiatric hospital. *In* "Assaults within Psychiatric Facilities". (Eds J.R. Lion and W.H. Reid), pp. 81-89. Grune and Stratton, Orlando, Florida.

Aiken, G.J.M. (1984). Assaults on staff in a locked ward: prediction and consequences. *Medicine, Science and the Law*, **24**, 199-207.

Armond, A.D. (1982). Violence in the semisecure ward of a psychiatric hospital. *Medicine, Science and the Law*, **22**, 203-209.

Blackburn, R. (1968a). Emotionality, extraversion and aggression of paranoid and non-paranoid offenders. *British Journal of Psychiatry,* **115**, 1301-1302.

Blackburn, R. (1968b). Personality in relation to extreme aggression in psychiatric offenders. *British Journal of Psychiatry,* **114**, 821-828.

Blackburn, R. (1987). Two scales for the assessment of personality in antisocial populations. *Personality and Individual Differences,* **8**, 81-93.

Blomhoff, S., Seim, S. and Friis, S. (1990). Can prediction of violence among psychiatry inpatients be improved? *Hospital and Community Psychiatry,* **41**, 771-775.

Brizer, D.A., Convit, A., Krakowski, M. and Volavka, J. (1987). A rating scale for reporting violence on psychiatric wards. *Hospital and Community Psychiatry,* **38**, 769-770.

Buss, A. and Durkee, A. (1957). An inventory for assessing different kinds of hostility. *Journal of Consulting and Clinical Psychology,* **4**, 343-349.

Carmel, H. and Hunter, M. (1989). Staff injuries from inpatient violence. *Hospital and Community Psychiatry,* **40**, 41-46.

Coldwell, J. and Naismaith, L. (1990). Violent incidents in special hospitals (letter). *British Journal of Psychiatry,* **154**, 270.

Conn, L.M. and Lion, J.R. (1983). Assaults in a University Hospital. *In* "Assaults within Psychiatric Facilities". (Eds J.R. Lion and W.H. Reid), pp. 61-69. Grune and Stratton, Orlando, Florida.

Convey, J. (1986). A record of violence. *Nursing Times,* 12/11/86, pp.36-38.

Convit, A., Isay, D., Gadioma, R. and Volavka, T. (1988a). Underreporting of physical assaults in schizophrenic inpatients. *Journal of Nervous and Mental Disease,* **176**, 507-509.

Convit, A., Jaeger, J., Pinlin, S., Meisner, M. and Volavka, J. (1988b). Predicting assaultiveness in psychiatric patients: a pilot study. *Hospital and Community Psychiatry,* **39**, 429-434.

Convit, A., Isay, D., Otis, D. and Volavka, J. (1990). Characteristics of repeatedly assaultive psychiatric patients. *Hospital and Community Psychiatry,* **41**, 1112-1115.

Cooper, S.J., Browne, F.W.A., McClean, K.J. *et al.* (1983). Aggressive behaviour in a psychiatric observation ward. *Acta Psychiatrica Scandinavica,* **68**, 386-393.

De Pauw, K. and Szulecka, K. (1988). Dangerous delusions. Violence and the misidentificantion syndromes. *British Journal of Psychiatry,* **152**, 91-96.

Drinkwater, J. (1982). Violence in psychiatric hospitals. *In* "Developments in the Study of Criminal Behaviour: Vol. 2. Violence". (Ed. P. Feldman), pp.111-130. Wiley, Chichester.

Edmunds, G. and Kendrick, D. (1980). "The Measurement of Human Aggression". Ellis Horwood, Chichester, England.

Edwards, A. (1954). "Manual for the Personal Preference Schedule". Psychological Corporation, New York.

Evans, D. and Strangeland, M. (1971). Development of the reaction inventory to measure anger. *Psychological Reports,* **29**, 412-414.

Eysenck H.J. and Eysenck, S.B. (1975). "Manual Eysenck Personality Questionnaire (Junior and Adult)". Edits, San Diego.

Fottrell, E. (1980). A study of violent behaviour among patients in psychiatric hospitals. *British Journal of Psychiatry,* **136**, 216-221.

Haller, R.M. and Deluty, R.H. (1988). Assaults on staff by psychiatric inpatients: a critical review. *British Journal of Psychiatry,* **152**, 174-179.

Hazaleus, S. and Deffenbacher, J. (1986). Relaxation and cognitive treatments of anger. *Journal of Consulting and Clinical Psychology,* **54**, 222-226.

Hellerstein, D., Frosch, W. and Konigsberg, H. (1987). The clinical significance of command hallucinations, *American Journal of Psychiatry,* **144**, 219-221.

Hinde, R. (1990). Aggression integration ethology and the social sciences. *In* "Violence and Suicidality". (Eds H.M. VanPragg, R. Plutchik and A. Apter). Brunner/Mazel, New York.

Hodgkinson, P.E., McIvor, L. and Philips, M. (1985). Patient assaults on staff in a psychiatric hospital: a 2 year retrospective study. *Medicine, Science and the Law,* **25**, 288-294.

Home Office (1983). "The British Crime Survey: first Report". HMSO, London.

Howell, K. and Hollin, C. (1989). "Clinical Approaches to Violence". John Wiley and Son, Chichester.

James, D.V., Fineberg, N.A., Shah, A.K. and Priest, (1990). An increase in violence on an acute psychiatric ward: a study of associated factors. *British Journal of Psychiatry,* **156**, 846-852.

Janofsky, J. S., Spears, S. and Neubauer, D.N. (1988). Psychiatrists' accuracy in predicting violent behaviour on an inpatient unit. *Hospital and Community Psychiatry,* **39**, 1090-1094.

Katz and Kirkland (1990). Violence and social structure on hospital wards. *Psychiatry,* **53**, 262-278.

Kay, S., Wolkenfield, F. and Murrill, L. (1988*a*). Profiles of aggression among psychiatric patients. I. Nature and prevalence, *Journal of Nervous and Mental Disease,* **176**, 539-546.

Kay, S., Wolkenfield, F. and Murrill, L. (1988*b*). Profiles of aggression among psychiatric patients. II. Covariates and predictors. *Journal of Nervous and Mental Disease,* **176**, 547-557.

Krakowski, M., Volavka, J. and Brizer, D. (1986). Psychopathology and violence: A review of the literature. *Comprehensive Psychiatry,* **27**, 131-148.

Lion, J.R., Snyder, W. and Merrill, G.L. (1981). Underreporting of assaults on staff in state hospitals. *Hospital and Community Psychiatry,* **32**, 497-498.

Lowenstein, M., Binder, R.L. and McNield. (1990). The relationship between admission symptoms and Hospital Assualts. *Hospital and Community Psychiatry,* **41**, 311-313.

McGurk, B. (1980). The validity and utility of a typology of homicides based on Megargee's theory of control. *Personality and Individual Differences,* 129-136.

Megargee, E. (1966). Undercontrolled and overcontrolled personality types in extreme anti-social aggression. *Psychological Monographs,* **80**, No. 611.

Megargee, E., Cook, P. and Mendelsohn, G. (1967). Development and validation of an MMPI scale of assaultiveness in overcontrolled individuals. *Journal of Abnormal Psychology,* **72**, 519-528.

Monahan, J. (1981). "Predicting Violent Behaviour: an Assessment of Clinical Techniques". Sage Publications, Beverley Hills, California.

Noble, P. and Rodgers, S. (1989). Violence by psychiatric inpatients. *British Journal of Psychiatry,* **155**, 384-390.

Novaco, R. (1975). "Anger Control: the Development and Evaluation of an Experimental Treatment". Lexington Books, Lexington LA.

Novaco, R. (1991). Anger and violence among state hospital patients. *Aggressive Behavior,* **17**, 88.

Palmstierna, T. and Wistedt, B. (1987). Staff observation aggression scales: Presentation and evaluation, *Acta Psychiatrica Scandinavica,* **76**, 657-663.

Palmstierna, T., Lassenius, R. and Wistedt, B. (1989). Evaluation of the brief psychopathological (*sic*) rating scale in relation to aggressive behaviour by acute involuntarily admitted patients. *Acta Psychiatrica Scandinavica,* **79**, 313-316.

Pearson, M., Wilmot, E. and Padi, M. (1986). A study of violent behaviour among inpatients in a psychiatric hospital. *British Journal of Psychiatry,* **149**, 232-235.

Planansky, K. and Johnson, R. (1977). Homicidal aggression in schizophrenic men. *Acta Psychiatrica Scandinavica,* **55**, 65-73.

Poster, E. C. and Ryan, J.A. (1989). Nurses attitudes towards physical assaults by patients. *Archives of Psychiatric Nursing,* **3**, 315-322.

Rabkin, J. (1979). Criminal behaviour of discharged mental patients: A critical appraisal of the research. *Psychological Bulletin,* **86**, 1-27.

Rogers, R. and Salvage, J. (1988). "Nurses at Risk: A Guide to Health and Safety at Work". Heinemann, London.

Selby, M. (1984). Assessment of violence potential using measures of Anger, Hostility and Social Desirability. *Journal of Personality Assessment,* **48**, 531-544.

Tanke, E. and Yesavage, J. (1985). Characteristics of assaultive patients who do not provide visible cues of potential violence. *American Journal of Psychiatry,* **142**, 1409-1413.

Taylor, P. (1985). Motives for offending among violent and psychotic men. *British Journal of Psychiatry,* **147**, 491-498.

Tedeschi, J., Smith, R. and Brown, C. (1974). A reinterpretation of research on aggression. *Psychological Bulletin,* **81**, 540-562.

Volavka, J. and Kline, N. (1989). Schizophrenia and violence. *Psychological Medicine,* **19**, 559-562.

Volavka, J. and Krakowski, M. (1989). Schizophrenia and violence. *Psychological Medicine,* **19**, 559-562.

Wamsley, R. (1986). "Personal Violence". Home Office Research and Policy Unit Research Study No. 89 HMSO, London.

Yesavage, J., Werner, P., Becker, J. *et al.* (1981). Inpatient evaluation of aggression in psychiatric patients. *Journal of Nervous and Mental Disease,* **169**, 299-302.

Yudofsky, S., Silver, J., Jackson, W. , Endicott, J. and Williams, D. (1986). The Overt Aggression Scale for the objective rating of verbal and physical aggression. *American Journal of Psychiatry,* **143**, 35-49.

Rating Instruments and Diagnostic Criteria Index

Index